Nursing Care

In

Alzheimer's unit

The Complete Guide

ALEXANDRE CAREWELL

Table of contents

« *We must not see Alzheimer's disease as a condemnation to the inevitable loss of memory and function, but as a disease that can be prevented and, one day, cured.* »

- Dr. Rudolph E. Tanzi.

Chapter 1:
INTRODUCTION
ALZHEIMER'S DISEASE

Definition and
characteristics ofthe disease

Alzheimer's disease, often referred to by the general public with an air of mystery about it, is in fact a neurodegenerative disease that takes root deep in the brain. It is the most common form of dementia, accounting for 60-80% of cases. But what exactly defines this disease?

At the heart of this disorder is a progressive weakening of the patient's cognitive functions. It often begins with simple forgetfulness or lapses of time, but this memory loss can quickly progress to more significant forgetfulness, affecting daily life. Next, the disease works its way into more complex abilities such as judgement, thinking and finally behaviour, personality and motor functions.

A journey through the brain of a person with Alzheimer's disease reveals amyloid plaques and neurofibrillary tangles. These abnormal structures hinder communication between neurons, causing them to die and the brain to progressively shrink. These physiological changes are silent witnesses to a storm raging within, affecting the way memories are formed, stored and recalled.

However, Alzheimer's disease is not an integral part of ageing, although it is more common in people aged 65 and over. There is also a rarer but equally pernicious form known as early-onset Alzheimer's, which can affect people as young as their forties.

The symptoms and progression of the disease can vary from person to person. For some, the decline may be slow and almost imperceptible for years, while for others it may be rapid and devastating. This spectrum of manifestations is one of the reasons why early diagnosis is crucial. Early diagnosis can not only help put coping strategies in place, but also open the door to treatments that, while not curing the disease, can slow its progression.

To this day, Alzheimer's remains a medical, social and human challenge. Despite advances in research, the exact causes remain a mystery, as does the search for a cure. But one thing is certain: understanding this disease means above all embracing the complexity of the human mind and the urgent need to protect our ability to remember, think and feel.

History and discovery

The historical roots of Alzheimer's disease go back to the beginning of the twentieth century, although the symptoms associated with dementia were known long before that. This is the story of a discovery, scientific collaboration and the gradual recognition of a disease that today bears the name of a German neurologist.

In 1901, in Frankfurt, Dr. Alois Alzheimer met a patient called Auguste Deter. She was 51 years old and had symptoms that were intriguing to say the least: profound memory loss, hallucinations and language disorders. Describing her condition, Auguste once said: *"I've lost myself"*. The rapid progression of her symptoms led to her death only five years later. Intrigued by his case, Alzheimer examined his brain post-mortem, venturing into the depths of his brain tissue.

What he discovered was revolutionary. Augustus' brain was riddled with plaques and tangles - the same amyloid plaques and neurofibrillary tangles that researchers now associate with the disease. In 1906, at a conference in Tübingen, Alzheimer presented his findings, highlighting these brain abnormalities and linking them to dementia.

However, despite this major discovery, it was not until the 1970s that Alzheimer's disease was recognised as the main cause of dementia. Prior to this, dementia was often seen as an inevitable consequence of ageing. It was with the accumulation of evidence, advances in neuroimaging techniques and increasing longevity that the distinction between normal ageing and Alzheimer's disease became clear.

Over the years, advances in research have led to a better understanding of the underlying biological mechanisms, genetic and environmental risk factors, and the clinical course of the disease. New theories have emerged, drugs have been developed, and prevention strategies have been explored.

Today, more than a century after Alzheimer's was first described, we are at the dawn of an unprecedented era of research and innovation. And although the fight against this disease remains a major challenge, the tireless efforts of researchers, doctors and carers offer hope of a future in which Alzheimer's disease could be controlled, or even eradicated.

Epidemiology and prevalence

Epidemiology, the science which studies the factors influencing health and disease in populations, gives us a panoramic view of the extent and distribution of Alzheimer's disease around the world. The prevalence of Alzheimer's disease in particular highlights not only its current societal impact, but also the challenges we will face in the future.

Alzheimer's disease affects tens of millions of people worldwide. In fact, it is estimated that one person develops the disease every three seconds. Although Alzheimer's disease is universal, affecting individuals from all regions and ethnic backgrounds, there are regional variations in terms of prevalence. These differences can be explained by genetic, environmental, cultural and even socio-economic factors.

Increased longevity, particularly in developed countries, is one of the main drivers of this rising prevalence. Age remains the most significant risk factor: the risk of developing the disease doubles every five years after the age of 65. What's more, as the world's elderly population increases, the absolute number of cases is set to rise exponentially. Some experts predict that, by 2050, more than 130 million people worldwide could be affected by Alzheimer's disease.

The epidemic is not just a phenomenon of developed countries. Low- and middle-income countries, where resources and infrastructures for diagnosing and treating dementia are often limited, are also experiencing a rapid increase in cases. In these regions, the disease is unfortunately often under-diagnosed, leading to additional challenges in terms of care and support.

There is also a difference in prevalence between the sexes. Women are more often affected by Alzheimer's disease than men. While some theories suggest that women live longer, others suggest that hormonal or genetic differences may play a role.

The epidemiology of Alzheimer's disease is therefore a reflection of our changing society, the challenges of an ageing population, and the urgent need for innovative solutions to prevent, treat and manage the disease. In this context, understanding the figures and trends is essential not only for researchers and healthcare professionals, but also for decision-makers, communities and families around the world.

Progression and stages of the disease

Alzheimer's disease, by its insidious nature and gradual progression, takes affected individuals on a journey where each stage presents its own challenges, symptoms and care needs. Understanding the stages of the disease is crucial to adapting care, anticipating future needs and providing the best possible support for patients and their families throughout this journey.

1. Pre-clinical stage (asymptomatic)
Even before the first symptoms appear, biological changes are taking place in the brain. Thanks to the development of brain imaging technologies and blood tests, it is now possible to detect these early signs, such as the accumulation of amyloid plaques. Although the person may not yet have cognitive problems, identifying this early stage opens the door to preventive interventions or participation in clinical trials.

2. Mild cognitive decline (MCI)

At this stage, symptoms become noticeable but remain relatively minor. The person may experience occasional memory loss, forget words or have difficulty performing certain tasks that used to be routine. However, these symptoms are not severe enough to interfere with daily activities and are not always recognised as signs of progression to Alzheimer's disease.

3. Mild Alzheimer's disease (initial stage)

The problems become more apparent and begin to affect daily life. Forgetfulness increases, and the person may get lost, have difficulty managing finances or following a conversation. Personality changes may also occur, such as social withdrawal or irritability.

4. Moderate Alzheimer's disease (intermediate stage)

This is the longest and often the most difficult stage. Cognitive abilities continue to deteriorate. The person may forget important events in their life, confuse family members or require help with activities of daily living such as dressing or bathing. Language problems, sleep disturbances and unpredictable behaviour may also occur.

5. Severe Alzheimer's disease (advanced stage)

At this stage, dependence is total. Memory has deteriorated significantly, and communication becomes extremely limited. Physical complications appear, such as difficulty swallowing or loss of mobility. Constant monitoring and care are required to ensure the patient's well-being.

Each stage of Alzheimer's disease presents unique challenges, but also opportunities to strengthen support, love and understanding for the person affected. Understanding these stages enables us to adapt our interventions, anticipate needs and offer personalised support throughout this ordeal.

Chapter 2:
THE ALZHEIMER'S UNIT:
A WORLD APART

The specific nature of
the Alzheimer's unit

When it comes to caring for people with Alzheimer's disease, the approach cannot be generic. The progression and complexity of the disease require a tailored, personalised and multidimensional response. It is with this in mind that the Alzheimer's units have been designed, offering an infrastructure, a philosophy of care and expertise specifically dedicated to this condition.

1. Design and environment
The Alzheimer's unit is first and foremost a place designed for the comfort and safety of residents. It minimises stimuli likely to cause confusion or agitation. The design is intuitive, with clearly defined pathways, soothing colours, appropriate lighting and clear signage to aid orientation. In addition, secure outdoor areas, such as therapeutic gardens, can be integrated, giving residents the opportunity to enjoy nature while being safe.

2. Person-centred approach
Far from being a "one size fits all" approach, each care plan is tailored to the individual. This takes into account the resident's life history, preferences, needs and residual abilities. By recognising the person behind the illness, the Alzheimer's unit aims to maintain the respect, dignity and well-being of each resident.

3. A multidisciplinary team

The professionals in these units are specifically trained in the care of Alzheimer's disease. They range from nurses and care assistants to occupational therapists, psychologists, neuropsychologists and physiotherapists. Each brings his or her own expertise to bear in providing holistic care, addressing cognitive, physical and emotional symptoms simultaneously.

4. Non-drug therapies

In addition to drug treatments, the Alzheimer's unit focuses on non-pharmacological interventions to enrich residents' lives and manage symptoms. These may include music therapy, art therapy, animal therapy, as well as relaxation and meditation techniques.

5. Support for families

Alzheimer's disease affects not only the individual, but also those around them. Alzheimer's units often offer information sessions, support groups and advice to help families understand, adapt and support their loved ones throughout the disease.

The specificity of the Alzheimer's unit lies in its integrative, person-centred approach, offering an environment and interventions adapted to the complexity of this disease. It aims not only to ensure the well-being of people with the disease, but also to support, educate and work hand in hand with families to provide the best possible quality of life for each resident.

The particular challenges of care in an Alzheimer's unit

The care of patients with Alzheimer's disease in specialist units, while focused on optimising well-being and safety, is fraught with pitfalls and challenges. These challenges reflect the complexities inherent in the disease itself, but also the societal, institutional and personal challenges faced by carers.

1. Difficult behaviour

Behavioural problems such as agitation, aggression, wandering and sleep disturbances are common in people with Alzheimer's disease. These behaviours can be stressful and demanding for the care team, requiring an empathetic, adaptive and sometimes creative approach to respond effectively.

2. Impaired communication

As the disease progresses, the patient's ability to communicate erodes, making it difficult to understand their needs and pass on information. For carers, this means developing skills in non-verbal communication and learning to 'read' the subtle clues in the patient's behaviour.

3. Burnout

Alzheimer's care is emotionally and physically demanding. Repetition, the emotional burden of patients' deterioration and the need for constant attention can lead to burn-out among carers.

4. Training and specialist skills

Not all healthcare professionals are equally trained to meet the specific needs of Alzheimer's patients. Specialised units require ongoing training and updates to ensure optimal care.

5. Ethical issues

Ethical issues often arise in healthcare. These questions may concern physical or chemical restraint, respect for patient autonomy in medical decisions, or the management of situations where patient safety conflicts with individual rights.

6. Family support

Families, often overwhelmed by the progress of their loved one's illness, seek support, information and sometimes guidance in making difficult decisions. Meeting these needs while managing direct care can be complex.

7. Resources and funding

Specialised care is expensive. Establishments face budgetary pressures, the need to maintain a sufficient number of qualified staff and to provide appropriate facilities and equipment.

8. Constantly evolving care

As research advances, new approaches, therapies and medicines may emerge. Units need to stay at the forefront of these developments to offer the best possible care.

While Alzheimer's units represent an essential response to the needs of people with the disease, they also raise a number of challenges. Recognising, understanding and working on these challenges is crucial to ensuring quality care, supporting carers and offering patients as fulfilling a life as possible, despite the disease.

The importance of a suitable environment

Caring for people with Alzheimer's disease is not based solely on medical or therapeutic interventions. The physical environment in which patients live plays a decisive role in their well-being, safety and, more broadly, in the quality of their daily lives. A suitable environment can considerably reduce some of the symptoms of the disease and help the sufferer to flourish.

1. Safety and risk prevention

Cognitive impairment can make people more vulnerable to accidents. A suitable environment minimises these risks by eliminating obstacles, making high-risk areas such as stairs or the bathroom safe, providing sufficient lighting to prevent falls, and installing warning devices.

2. Guidance and autonomy

Disorientation is common among people with Alzheimer's disease. Clear, legible design makes orientation easier: use of contrasting colours, simple signage, clearly defined spaces and familiar landmarks. All this helps people to move around with greater independence and confidence.

3. Controlled stimulation

Too many stimuli can be a source of confusion or agitation. It is essential to strike a balance: a calm environment, soothing colours, controlled acoustics, while offering areas where the person can interact, such as a sensory garden or areas dedicated to activities.

4. Memories and continuity

Incorporating familiar or evocative items from the past can provide anchors for the ill person: family photos, everyday objects, favourite music. These points of reference can soothe, reassure and help connect with memories.

5. Flexibility

The progression of the disease fluctuates and varies from person to person. A suitable environment is one that can evolve to meet the patient's changing needs, whether in terms of mobility, cognitive abilities or behaviour.

6. Social spaces

Alzheimer's disease can lead to isolation. Spaces dedicated to socialising encourage interaction, whether with other residents, staff or family. These spaces foster a sense of belonging and help maintain social skills.

7. Close to nature

Numerous studies have shown the benefits of contact with nature on psychological well-being. Secure gardens, patios or even simple views of green spaces can have a positive impact on mood and reduce problem behaviour.

8. Support for family and carers

A well-designed environment also facilitates the work of carers, by reducing risks and promoting better care. What's more, dedicated areas can be set aside for families to spend quality time with their loved ones.

The importance of a suitable environment in Alzheimer's disease cannot be underestimated. More than just a living environment, it is a therapeutic tool in itself, aimed at maximising the well-being and dignity of each person, while supporting those who care for them.

Chapter 3:
THE ESSENTIAL ROLE OF THE NURSE

A vocation focused on people

Behind every diagnosis of Alzheimer's disease lies a person with his or her own story, dreams, joys, fears and aspirations. More than just a medical approach focused on the disease, Alzheimer's care requires a resolutely person-centred approach. This perspective highlights the dignity and intrinsic value of each individual, far beyond the symptoms of the disease.

1. Recognising uniqueness
Every person with Alzheimer's is unique. Their experiences, their relationships and their passions all form the prism through which they perceive and interact with the world. So rather than seeing a patient, carers strive to see a rich and full life.

2. Listening and communication
Even if the illness affects the ability to communicate, this does not mean that the person has nothing to say. Listening actively, paying attention to what is left unsaid, seeking to understand beyond the words, means respecting the voice and desire of the person who is ill.

3. The right to autonomy
As long as possible, it is essential to let the person make decisions about their life and care. This may involve day-to-day choices, such as what to wear, or more substantial decisions about treatment.

4. Maintaining identity
Alzheimer's disease can erode memory and self-perception, but this does not mean that the person's identity is gone. Carers should strive to recall and reinforce

this identity, whether through stories, photos, music or other memories.

5. Relationships and human connection
Social ties remain crucial. Cultivating relationships and encouraging interaction with family, friends and even other residents means giving people the opportunity to feel, love and be loved.

6. Respect and dignity
Despite the challenges posed by illness, every individual deserves respect and dignity in all aspects of their care. This means caring for the person as a whole individual, considering their physical, emotional, social and spiritual needs.

7. Holistic approach
Person-centred care embraces all aspects of the human being. It involves not only treating symptoms, but also nourishing the mind, stimulating the senses, soothing the emotions and encouraging social interaction.

The person-centred approach to Alzheimer's care is an ethical and human imperative. It recognises and values the humanity of each person, ensuring that, despite the progression of the disease, the light of the individual continues to shine with dignity, respect and love.

Communication techniques with the Alzheimer patient

Communicating with someone who has Alzheimer's disease can be a challenge due to the cognitive impairments associated with the disease. However, effective communication is essential to understanding the patient's needs, offering comfort and maintaining a meaningful relationship. Here are some techniques for facilitating communication with Alzheimer's patients:

1. Adopt a calm and patient attitude
Always start the conversation with a relaxed approach. Your calmness can help to ease the patient's anxiety or confusion.

2. Make eye contact
Before you speak, make sure you've made eye contact. This attracts the person's attention and strengthens the connection between you.

3. Use simple language
Opt for short, simple sentences, avoiding complicated turns of phrase. Ask direct questions that require short answers, such as *"Would you like some tea?"* rather than open-ended questions.

4. Avoid distractions
Minimise background noise and other distractions when communicating. This can include turning down the volume on the television or choosing a quiet environment.

5. Using non-verbal language
Body language, facial expressions and touch can sometimes communicate more than words. A reassuring smile or a gentle hand on the shoulder can offer comfort and understanding.

6. Validate rather than correct
If the patient evokes memories that seem inaccurate or experiences hallucinations, it is often more beneficial to validate their feelings rather than correct them. For example, rather than saying, *"Your mother died a long time ago,"* you might say, *"Tell me more about your mother."*

7. Listen actively
Show that you are listening and that you care about what they are saying, even if it may seem rambling or difficult to follow. The simple fact of feeling heard can have a huge impact on a patient's well-being.

8. Repeat or rephrase as necessary
If the patient seems confused, gently repeat or rephrase your question or statement.

9. Use visual aids
Photos, familiar objects or other visual aids can help to stimulate memory or facilitate understanding.

10. Preserving dignity
Even if communication becomes difficult, it is essential to treat the person with Alzheimer's with respect and dignity. Avoid talking about them as if they weren't there or infantilising them.

11. Remembering the good times
Recalling pleasant memories or special moments can create a connection and encourage positive communication.

12. Adjust as you go
An Alzheimer's patient's ability to communicate can vary from day to day. Be flexible and adapt to the patient's condition at the time.

The key is to approach communication with empathy, patience and openness. Even though Alzheimer's disease can impair the ability to communicate, the fundamental need for connection, understanding and respect remains.

Specific treatments and standard procedures

Care for Alzheimer's patients is not limited to addressing the cognitive symptoms of the disease. Care is multidimensional, encompassing the patient's physical, emotional, social and sometimes spiritual needs. In an Alzheimer's unit, the following are some of the specific care and procedures commonly practised:

1. Regular cognitive assessment
Progression of the disease is monitored by repeated cognitive assessments, often using standardised tools.

2. Medication management
Polypharmacy (the use of numerous medications) is common among the elderly. It is essential to monitor the drugs used to treat Alzheimer's symptoms and other concomitant medical conditions.

3. Skin care
Patients may be less mobile, increasing the risk of pressure ulcers. Regular attention is paid to the condition of the skin, with frequent changes of position and the use of moisturisers or barriers.

4. Nutrition and hydration
Alzheimer's disease can disrupt a person's sense of hunger or thirst. Carers help with feeding, monitor food and fluid intake, and may use specialised diets or food supplements.

5. Non-drug therapies
Interventions such as music therapy, art therapy or animal therapy can be beneficial for mood, cognition and general well-being.

6. Daily hygiene care
This includes bathing, hair care, brushing the teeth and cutting the nails. These routines are essential not only for physical health but also for personal dignity.

7. Physiotherapy and exercise
Maintaining mobility and strength can help prevent falls and improve quality of life. Exercises can be adapted to each individual's abilities.

8. End-of-life care
As the disease progresses, discussions and care focused on comfort, pain and end-of-life preferences become paramount.

9. Psychosocial support
The unit's social worker or psychologist can offer emotional support to the patient and their family, helping to manage the psychological challenges associated with the illness.

10. Preventing and managing problem behaviour
Behaviours such as agitation, aggression or wandering may be common. Interventions include non-medication strategies, environmental modifications and, if necessary, medication.

11. Stimulating activities
Adapted daily activities, such as gardening, puzzles or reading, can help stimulate cognition and provide a sense of purpose.

12. Training and support for families
Families often receive training on the disease, how to communicate effectively, and how to manage the challenges at home.

As each patient is unique, the key to effective care in an Alzheimer's unit lies in an individualised, adaptive and empathetic approach. Caregivers work closely together to provide holistic care that encompasses all aspects of the patient's health and well-being.

Chapter 4:
MULTIDISCIPLINARY COLLABORATION

Work with a diverse medical team

Working in an Alzheimer's unit requires a multidisciplinary approach. Each member of the team plays a crucial role in the overall care of the patient, and effective collaboration between specialities ensures quality care. Let's look at the dynamics of working in a diverse medical team in an Alzheimer's unit:

1. Composition of the team
The typical team in an Alzheimer's unit generally comprises :

- **Doctors**: Geriatricians or neurologists specialising in the management of neurodegenerative disorders.
- **Nurses**: They are often the first line of care, providing direct care, administering medication and monitoring patients' general condition.
- **Care assistants**: They provide essential assistance with daily activities, such as hygiene, eating and mobility.
- **Psychologists or psychiatrists**: They offer support for the emotional and behavioural challenges associated with the disease.
- **Therapists**: Physiotherapists, occupational therapists, speech therapists and others, who offer tailored therapies.
- **Social workers**: They offer support to families and refer them to the appropriate resources or services.
- **Leisure staff**: They plan and implement appropriate activities to stimulate and engage patients.

2. Open communication
Clear and open communication between team members is essential to ensure consistency of care. Regular team meetings provide an opportunity to discuss challenges, care plans and updates on patients' condition.

3. Complementary roles
Each professional brings specific expertise to the table, and mutual recognition of these skills promotes holistic patient care.

4. Further training
The rapid development of knowledge about Alzheimer's disease requires ongoing training for the team. Training sessions, workshops and conferences are essential to keep the team up to date.

5. Conflict management
As in any team, disagreements can arise. Proactive conflict management, based on mutual respect and listening, is crucial.

6. Emotional support within the team
Working in an Alzheimer's unit can be emotionally challenging. It is therefore vital to have support mechanisms in place for professionals, whether in the form of debriefing sessions, supervision or advice.

7. Family involvement
The medical team works closely with families, often regarding them as "care partners". This collaboration makes it possible to obtain valuable information about the patient and to offer appropriate support to the family.

The success of care in Alzheimer's units depends on a close-knit team, where each member is valued for their expertise. Harmonious collaboration ensures that every aspect of the patient's health and well-being is taken into account, providing the best possible care.

The importance of collaboration for comprehensive care

Because of its complexity and multiple dimensions, Alzheimer's disease requires a collaborative approach to provide holistic and effective care. This collaboration transcends mere professional interaction to become the very heart of the therapeutic approach. Here's why collaboration is so essential:

1. Complexity of the disease
Alzheimer's disease is more than just a memory problem. It affects behaviour, emotions, communication, motor skills and much more. To meet this wide range of needs, a multidisciplinary team is essential.

2. Integrated care design
Care for Alzheimer's patients cannot be segmented. The intervention of one professional may have an impact on another aspect of the patient's well-being. For example, a change in medication may influence a patient's ability to participate in physical therapy. Collaboration ensures that these interdependent implications are taken into account.

3. Complete patient perspective
While a neurologist may focus on the neurological progression of the disease, a social worker can provide insights into the social and family challenges faced by the patient. Together, these varied perspectives provide a holistic understanding of the patient's situation.

4. Continuity of care

Constant communication and collaboration between professionals ensures that care is continuous and consistent, with no overlaps or gaps.

5. Enhancing therapeutic efficacy

When therapists, nurses, doctors and other professionals work hand in hand, interventions can be harmonised to maximise their impact. For example, an occupational therapy session can be planned in synergy with the patient's medication regime to optimise attention and concentration.

6. Mutual support

Caring for Alzheimer's patients can be emotionally demanding. Working closely together allows team members to support each other, sharing challenges and successes.

7. Education and training

A collaborative team offers opportunities for mutual learning. Nurses can learn more about the latest therapeutic interventions, while therapists can better understand the medical implications of treatments.

8. Involvement of family and friends

Family and friends are key partners in care. By incorporating their observations, concerns and needs into the collaborative care plan, the team can offer more personalised and sensitive care.

Collaboration is not just a beneficial aspect of care in an Alzheimer's unit; it is absolutely vital. Only close and harmonious collaboration can ensure that every aspect of the patient's life is considered, valued and cared for in the best possible way.

Key players:
psychologists, physiotherapists, occupational therapists, etc.

Within an Alzheimer's unit, various specialist professionals are involved, each contributing to a specific aspect of care. Together, they form a coherent team, focused on the well-being and quality of life of patients. Find out more about the roles and contributions of these key players.

1. Psychologists
- **Role**: Psychologists provide emotional and behavioural support to patients and their families.
    - Contribution :
    - Assessment of cognitive disorders and associated deficits.
    - Implementing strategies to manage the behavioural and psychological symptoms of dementia.
    - Providing psycho-educational support for families and loved ones.
    - Running workshops or support groups.

2. Physiotherapists (or physiotherapists)
- **Role**: These professionals work on patients' mobility, strength and balance.
    - Contribution :
    - Assessment of mobility and physical function.
    - Development of tailored exercise programmes to maintain or improve muscle strength and coordination.
    - Falls prevention and safety education.
    - Provision of treatments to manage joint pain or stiffness.

3. Occupational therapists
- **Role**: Occupational therapists help patients to maintain or regain their independence in activities of daily living.
    - Contribution :
    - Assessment of the patient's functional abilities in their environment.
    - Proposing environmental modifications to promote independence and safety.
    - Teaching compensatory strategies to make everyday tasks easier.
    - Assessment and adaptation of technical aids.

4. Speech therapists
- **Role**: Speech and language therapists focus on communication and swallowing disorders.
    - Contribution :
    - Assessment of language, speech and swallowing disorders.
    - Setting up rehabilitation programmes and strategies to improve or maintain communication skills.
    - Advice on communication aids and training for relatives.

5. Social workers
- **Role**: They provide support to patients and their families, helping them to navigate the healthcare system and access resources.
    - Contribution :
    - Assessment of social and family needs.
    - Referral to appropriate resources or services.
    - Support with administrative and legal procedures related to the illness.

6. Dieticians
  - **Role**: Dieticians assess and advise on patients' nutritional needs.
      - Contribution :
      - Assessment of eating habits and nutritional status.
      - Developing appropriate diets.
      - Educating patients and their families about nutrition.

These professionals, with their specialist skills, enrich the overall care provided in Alzheimer's units. Their collaboration is essential to meet the complex and interdependent needs of patients, guaranteeing coherent, adapted and person-centred care.

Chapter 5:
THERAPEUTIC APPROACH: BEYOND DRUGS

Non-pharmacological therapies and their effectiveness

Given the complexity and progression of Alzheimer's disease, non-pharmacological approaches play a vital role. These interventions are designed to improve quality of life, slow cognitive decline and manage the behavioural and psychological symptoms associated with the disease. Here is an overview of some of these therapies and their effectiveness.

1. Cognitive behavioural therapy (CBT)
   - **Description**: This is a form of psychotherapy that aims to change negative patterns of thought and behaviour.
   - **Effectiveness**: CBT can help manage anxiety, depression and certain problem behaviours associated with dementia.
2. Cognitive stimulation
   - **Description**: This encompasses a variety of activities designed to stimulate mental functioning.
   - **Effectiveness**: Cognitive stimulation has demonstrated modest but significant improvements in the overall cognitive functioning of people with Alzheimer's disease.
3. Music therapy
   - **Description**: Using music to evoke memories, emotions and interaction.

- **Effectiveness**: Music can reduce symptoms of agitation, anxiety and depression, while improving mood and social well-being.

4. Animal therapy
   - **Description**: The integration of animals, generally dogs or cats, as part of therapeutic care.
   - **Effectiveness**: This approach has been associated with a reduction in agitation, aggression and depression.

5. Reality orientation therapy
   - **Description**: Technique that seeks to anchor people in time, place and person.
   - **Effectiveness**: Can improve awareness of reality, emotional well-being and certain aspects of cognitive functioning.

6. Validation therapy
   - **Description**: An approach that seeks to validate the feelings and experiences of people with Alzheimer's, even if they do not correspond to objective reality.
   - **Effectiveness**: Can reduce stress and agitation and improve communication.

7. Art therapy
   - **Description**: Using different art forms as a means of expression.
   - **Effectiveness**: Promotes emotional expression, reduces agitation and can improve self-esteem.

8. Physical activity and exercise
   - **Description**: Exercise programmes adapted to improve strength, balance and mobility.
   - **Effectiveness**: Can slow cognitive decline, improve mood and reduce the risk of falls.

9. Light therapy
   - **Description**: Exposure to intense light to regulate the sleep-wake cycle.
   - **Effectiveness**: Can improve sleep disorders and nocturnal agitation.

Although these therapies have shown benefits for many patients, it is important to note that effectiveness varies from person to person. The key is an individualised approach, tailored to the specific needs and preferences of each patient. A combination of pharmacological and non-pharmacological interventions is often the most beneficial in holistically managing the challenges posed by Alzheimer's disease.

Music and art therapy
and other innovative methods

The world of Alzheimer's care has seen the emergence of a number of innovative therapies that move away from traditional approaches to offer alternative and enriching avenues of communication and expression. These modalities, with their emphasis on creativity and the senses, have the power to touch patients deeply, often where words alone may fail.

Music therapy
- **Description**: Music therapy uses music to address physical, emotional, cognitive and social needs. It may involve listening, creating or moving in rhythm.
    - Benefits :
    - Improved cognition and memory.
    - Reduction in agitated or aggressive behaviour.
    - Stimulation of deep emotional memories.
    - Strengthening social links and interaction.

Art therapy
- **Description**: Art therapy offers patients a means of visual expression, often through drawing, painting or sculpture.
    - Benefits :
    - Improved communication and emotional expression.

- Improving dexterity and coordination.
- Offers a sense of achievement and self-esteem.
- Provides a soothing distraction from symptoms and stress.

Movement and dance therapy

- **Description**: This modality encourages bodily movement as a means of expression and well-being.
  - Benefits :
  - Improved mobility and coordination.
  - Strengthening cardiovascular capacity.
  - Increased emotional well-being and reduced stress.
  - Promotes socialisation and collaboration.

Aromatherapy

- **Description**: Aromatherapy uses essential oils to stimulate the senses and promote relaxation.
  - Benefits :
  - Can reduce agitation and anxiety.
  - Promotes better sleep.
  - Can improve mood and energy.

Gardening therapy

- **Description**: Therapeutic gardening involves planting and caring for plants.
  - Benefits :
  - Encourages fine motor skills and coordination.
  - A feeling of connection with nature.
  - Promotes relaxation and stress reduction.

Virtual reality therapy

- **Description**: The use of technology to create immersive and stimulating environments.
  - Benefits :
  - Can help reliving and cognitive stimulation.
  - Provides enriching and entertaining experiences.
  - Encourages exploration and discovery.

Each of these modalities offers a unique and specific approach to the needs of Alzheimer's patients. The key is flexibility and adaptability: each patient is unique, and what works for one may not work for another. These therapies, by their holistic and person-centred nature, allow for individualised care that values and celebrates each individual, despite the challenges posed by the disease.

Cognitive stimulation: games, activities and techniques

Cognitive stimulation plays a crucial role in the care of people with Alzheimer's disease. It aims to maintain and improve cognitive function, reduce cognitive decline and promote a better quality of life. This set of activities is designed to engage and challenge the mind, focusing on preserved abilities rather than deficits.

1. Memory games
   - **Examples**: card games, memory games, image association games.
   - **Objective: To** encourage short-term memory, attention and visual recognition.
2. Puzzles and brainteasers
   - **Examples**: Simple puzzles with large pieces, logic games.
   - **Objective:** Strengthen problem solving, fine motor skills and hand-eye coordination.
3. Artistic activities
   - **Examples**: Drawing, painting, modelling.
   - **Objective: To** encourage creativity, emotional expression and dexterity.
4. Reading and writing exercises
   - **Examples**: Reading aloud, writing in newspapers, completing simple crosswords.

- **Objective: To** maintain language, comprehension and written expression.

5. Word games and board games
   - **Examples**: Scrabble, Bingo, riddles.
   - **Objective: To** stimulate vocabulary, critical thinking and socialisation.
6. Musical activities
   - **Examples**: Singing, listening to familiar songs, using simple instruments.
   - **Objective**: Strengthen memory, emotional expression and coordination.
7. Gentle physical exercise
   - **Examples**: Tai-chi, yoga, guided walking.
   - **Objective: To** improve coordination, strength, balance and general well-being.
8. Activities of daily living (ADL)
   - **Examples**: Folding laundry, setting the table, gardening.
   - **Objective**: Maintain independence, fine motor skills and a sense of achievement.
9. Sensory activities
   - **Examples**: sensory kits, touch bags, aromatherapy.
   - **Objective**: Stimulate the senses, promote relaxation and awareness of the environment.
10. Use of technology
    - **Examples**: Applications for tablets, adapted video games, virtual reality.
    - **Objective**: Offer a variety of cognitive challenges, improve coordination and visual recognition.

The success of these activities depends on their adaptability. The approach must be individualised, taking into account each person's cognitive level, interests and abilities. In addition, regularity is essential: regular cognitive stimulation can offer longer-lasting and more significant benefits. Finally, it is crucial that these activities are carried out in an encouraging environment, where successes are celebrated and challenges are tackled with patience and understanding.

Chapter 6:
MANAGING BEHAVIOURAL SYMPTOMS

Understanding behavioural manifestations

In people with Alzheimer's disease, behavioural changes can occur that are often unpredictable, making their management more complex. These behavioural manifestations are influenced by a combination of factors linked to the disease itself, as well as the patient's experiences and environment. Understanding these behaviours is essential to providing appropriate and empathetic care.

1. Agitation
Agitation may manifest itself as repetitive movements, increased anxiety or resistance to care.
- **Possible causes**: Pain, discomfort, fatigue, over-stimulation, frustration, changes in environment.
- **Recommended approach**: Identify and resolve the underlying cause, offer soothing activities, avoid over-stimulation, use reassuring communication.

2. Aggression
This can include shouting, sudden gestures or even acts of violence.
- **Possible causes**: Pain, fear, frustration, feelings of incomprehension.
- **Recommended approach**: Assess the situation calmly, ensure everyone's safety, use de-escalation techniques, avoid confrontation.

3. Repeat

Constantly repeating phrases, questions or actions is common.

- **Possible causes:** Short-term memory loss, need for structure, anxiety.
- **Recommended approach**: Provide short, reassuring answers, divert attention, use visual reminders.

4. Wandering

The person may appear to be wandering aimlessly.

- **Possible causes**: Disorientation, looking for something or someone, need for exercise.
- **Recommended approach**: Ensure a safe environment, offer structured activities, use safety devices.

5. Reactions to hallucinations or delusions

The patient can perceive things that are not really there.

- **Possible causes**: Changes to the brain, side effects of medication, infections.
- **Recommended approach**: Don't argue about reality, offer reassurance, assess medication and general health.

6. Reluctance to care

Resistance to or refusal of certain activities, such as toileting or dressing, is common.

- **Possible causes**: Pain, fear, loss of dignity, loss of understanding of the steps involved.
- **Recommended approach**: Simplify routines, encourage autonomy, offer choices, use a progressive approach.

7. Sleep disturbances

Changes in sleep patterns, such as night-time wakefulness, may occur.

- **Possible causes**: Temporal disorientation, side effects of medication, lack of exercise.
- **Recommended approach**: Establish a sleep routine, limit daytime naps, ensure a comfortable sleep environment.

8. Social misappropriation
Behaviours such as undressing in public or inappropriate language may appear.
- **Possible causes**: Loss of inhibition, confusion, physical discomfort.
- **Recommended approach**: Respond calmly, redirect behaviour, ensure privacy during personal care.

Understanding these behavioural manifestations requires a holistic approach. Beyond the visible symptoms, it is crucial to consider the whole person, taking into account their history, emotions and needs. Such an understanding can lead to more effective interventions and a better quality of life for patients.

Interventions and techniques for crisis management

Managing behavioural crises in Alzheimer's patients is one of the most demanding challenges for healthcare staff. These situations, which are often unpredictable, require rapid, effective and empathetic intervention. Here are some tried and tested techniques and interventions for dealing with these crises.

1. Rapid initial assessment
Before intervening, quickly assess the situation.

- **Objective**: To determine the immediate cause of the crisis and assess any potential danger to the patient or others.
- **Technique**: Observe, listen and interpret behaviour and the environment.

2. Ensuring safety

Safety is paramount.

- **Objective**: Prevent injuries.
- **Technique**: Keep all potentially dangerous objects away, make sure the area is secure and that the patient is physically stable.

3. Calm, reassuring communication

The way you communicate can make or break a crisis.

- **Objective**: De-escalate the situation.
- **Technique**: Use a gentle tone, simple, clear language, maintain friendly eye contact and avoid threatening body language.

4. Redirection and distraction

Diverting the patient's attention can interrupt undesirable behaviour.

- **Objective**: to channel the patient's energy into a positive activity.
- **Technique**: Suggest a pleasant or familiar activity, such as listening to music or going for a walk.

5. Emotional validation

Acknowledging the patient's emotions without judgement.

- **Objective**: Build rapport and show empathy.
- **Technique**: Express that you understand their feelings, even if you don't validate the distorted reality.

6. Reassessment of needs
Crises can often be the result of unmet needs.
- **Objective**: To identify and resolve underlying problems.
- **Technique**: Check for basic needs such as hunger, thirst, the need to use the toilet, or physical discomfort.

7. Minimal use of restraint
Physical or chemical restraint should be the last resort.
- **Objective**: Use only if the patient is a threat to themselves or others and if other methods have failed.
- **Technique**: Make sure you are properly trained, follow established protocols and constantly monitor the patient.

8. Post-crisis: Debriefing
After a crisis, it's essential to reflect on what happened.
- **Objective**: Prevent future crises.
- **Technique**: Assess triggers, discuss with the care team, and adjust care plans accordingly.

9. Continuing training
The world of dementia is constantly evolving, as are the best practices for its management.
- **Objective**: To keep up to date with the most effective techniques.
- **Technique**: Regularly take part in training courses, workshops and seminars on the care of Alzheimer's patients.

10. Support for staff
Crisis management can be emotionally draining for carers.
- **Objective: To** ensure the mental and emotional well-being of carers.

- **Technique**: Offer support sessions, regular debriefings and mental health resources.

Crisis management for Alzheimer's patients is as much an art as a science. As well as technical skills, humanity, patience and empathy are essential to providing appropriate and caring care.

Trigger factors and prevention of defiant behaviour

Managing defiant behaviour in Alzheimer's patients requires an in-depth understanding of the factors that can trigger these behaviours. Identifying and understanding these triggers is essential if effective preventive measures are to be put in place.

Common triggers:

1. Unmet physiological needs: Hunger, thirst, the need to go to the toilet or pain can cause agitation or frustration.

2. Overstimulating environment: Too much noise, bright light or large numbers of people can create confusion or stress.

3. Disruption of routine: People with Alzheimer's often rely on predictable routines. Any change can be destabilising.

4. Sensation of threat: New environments, new faces or an erroneous perception can lead to a feeling of danger.

5. Failure to communicate: A lack of understanding or an inability to express oneself can lead to frustration.

6. Medication: The side effects of certain drugs or drug interactions can influence behaviour.

7. Underlying health problems: Infections, constipation or other medical problems can alter behaviour without it being immediately obvious.

8. Fatigue: A lack of sleep or over-stimulation can accentuate defiant behaviour.

Prevention strategies:
1. Establish a routine: A predictable daily schedule can provide a sense of security.
2. Adapt the environment: Reduce sources of over-stimulation and create a safe, soothing environment.
3. Encourage clear communication: Use short sentences, gestures and visual aids to facilitate understanding.
4. Regularly assess physiological needs: Make sure the patient is well nourished, hydrated and pain-free.
5. Supervise medication: Regularly review medication to avoid undesirable side effects.
6. Participate in meaningful activities: Activities adapted to their abilities, such as music or the arts, can offer a sense of achievement.
7. Provide training for carers: Train staff and carers to recognise and respond to triggers for challenging behaviour.
8. Ensuring quality sleep: Establish a regular bedtime routine and ensure that the environment is conducive to sleep.

Preventing defiant behaviour in Alzheimer's patients requires constant attention and adaptability on the part of carers. The key lies in anticipating the patient's needs, adapting the environment and providing ongoing training to respond effectively to the challenges that arise.

Chapter 7:
RELATIONS WITH FAMILIES

Supporting relatives: a crucial mission

Alzheimer's disease does not just affect the patient. It also has a profound impact on those close to the person with the disease, be they family members, friends or carers. They live with the grief of seeing a loved one decline, while coping with the day-to-day challenges of caring for them. Supporting these individuals is essential, as they play a decisive role in the patient's well-being.

1. Recognising the role of family and friends
The importance of loved ones: Carers and family members are often the first to recognise symptoms and seek help. They provide constant support, adapting their daily lives to meet the patient's needs.

2. Education and information
Providing resources: Relatives need to be informed about the disease, its symptoms, its progression and best care practices. Workshops, books and information sessions can provide valuable tools.

3. Creating space for emotions
Acknowledging grief and loss: It is essential to create spaces where loved ones can express their feelings, share their experiences and receive emotional support.

4. Providing resources for well-being
Psychological support: Offer sessions with psychologists or specialist support groups. These can help loved ones deal with stress, anxiety and grief.

5. Easing the burden
Respite care: It is essential to give carers breaks to rest and recharge their batteries. This respite care can be provided by trained professionals or volunteers.

6. Involving relatives in the care plan
Joint planning: Actively involving family members in decisions about care ensures better understanding and appropriate care.

7. Preparation for subsequent steps
Early discussions: It is essential to discuss difficult issues, such as advance directives, end-of-life care and succession, with loved ones well before they become urgent.

8. Recognising family members as partners
Establishing solid links: Healthcare professionals need to establish a relationship of trust with relatives, recognising their essential role and valuing their contribution.

Alzheimer's care is a collective responsibility. By actively supporting family and friends, we can strengthen the chain of care around the patient, ensuring a loving and caring environment for all.

Educating families and raising awareness

When someone is diagnosed with Alzheimer's disease, it sends shockwaves through not only the life of the person affected, but also that of the whole family. Fear, uncertainty and lack of knowledge can quickly become the daily companions of loved ones. In this context, educating and raising awareness among families becomes essential.

Understanding Alzheimer's disease is more than just knowing the symptoms or anticipating its progression. Above all, it means grasping the profound upheaval it causes in the daily lives of patients and their families. It's vital to deconstruct preconceived ideas, demystify the disease and help people understand that, despite the changes, a person's identity and dignity remain.

Every family has its own history, dynamics, strengths and weaknesses. By raising awareness and educating each family according to its needs, we give them the tools they need to cope with this ordeal. Learning to communicate with someone suffering from Alzheimer's means relearning to connect in a different way, to focus on non-verbal communication, to look for the person behind the illness and to savour the moments of lucidity.

But this education would not be complete without preparing families for the different stages of the disease. Anticipation is essential if they are to adapt better. Although each patient's experience of the disease may be different, there are certain points of reference that families can use to prepare themselves, adjust their approach and draw on for better support for their loved one.

Finally, raising awareness and educating families also means reminding them that they are not alone. Exchanging with other families, joining support groups and taking part in workshops can all be lifesavers in this tumultuous situation. Solidarity, sharing experiences and mutual support are bulwarks against isolation and exhaustion.

In short, educating and raising awareness among families about Alzheimer's disease means reaching out to them, accompanying them on this winding road and reminding them that, despite the ordeals, love, patience and understanding remain the pillars on which to build.

Managing expectations and the emotions of families

Managing the expectations and emotions of families faced with Alzheimer's disease is one of the most delicate and essential aspects of patient support. The emotional turmoil generated by the diagnosis, and then by the progression of the disease, requires a gentle, understanding approach that seeks to anchor families in a reality they can understand and influence.

When Alzheimer's disease is diagnosed, it often bursts into the lives of families like an unwelcome intruder. It brings with it fears and anxieties, as well as sometimes exaggerated expectations about how the disease will progress or about possible treatments. In their search for answers, families can oscillate between denial, hope for a miracle cure and resignation.

Managing these expectations does not mean stifling hope, but rather channelling it in constructive directions. It means providing families with clear, factual information, educating them about what they can really expect from the progression of the disease and the treatments currently available. While this clarity may be painful at first, it has the merit of creating a stable foundation on which families can build their resilience.

As well as managing expectations, navigating the whirlwind of emotions is an equally complex task. Anger, sadness, guilt, despair and frustration are just some of the emotions that those close to a person with Alzheimer's may feel. While these emotions are natural, they can sometimes become obstacles if they are not recognised, accepted and dealt with.

It is therefore vital to have spaces where families can express their emotions and feelings without judgement. These spaces, whether they take the form of individual therapy, support groups or even creative workshops, offer a breath of fresh air, a place to share and listen.

In addition, strengthening communication within the family is essential. Encouraging dialogue between family members not only enables them to express their own emotions, but also to understand those of others, creating solidarity in the face of adversity.

In the end, by addressing the expectations and emotions of families together, we give them the means to make the best of this ordeal. In doing so, we remind them that in the midst of the storm, there are always moments of respite, moments of joy to be seized and cherished, even in the shadow of Alzheimer's disease.

Chapter 8:
TAKING CARE OF YOURSELF
AS A NURSE

Recognising and managing burnout

Recognising and dealing with burnout among relatives of people with Alzheimer's disease is crucial. This burnout syndrome, characterised by profound fatigue, diminished self-esteem and distancing from work or the people being cared for, can affect anyone involved in a caring role, whether a professional or a family member.

Caring for someone with Alzheimer's disease means total dedication. The days are the same, punctuated by routines, needs and crises. The nights can be short, interrupted by sudden awakenings. The emotional challenge is great: seeing a loved one forget, lose themselves, change, can be heartbreaking. In this context, burnout is just around the corner.

Recognising the warning signs of burnout is the first step in dealing with it. Persistent fatigue, increasing irritability, a feeling of being overwhelmed, a loss of interest in activities that used to be enjoyed, or a tendency to isolate yourself can be warning signs.

Managing burnout requires awareness and proactive action. Accepting the idea that, as a carer, you are not infallible is fundamental. It's crucial to set aside time to take a break and breathe, however briefly. Taking time out for yourself, whether to do something you enjoy, rest, meditate or simply go for a walk. It's when you recharge your batteries that you find the energy to continue supporting your loved one.

Those around you have a vital role to play. Sharing responsibilities, setting up a relay, or simply recognising the effort made can be a breath of fresh air for the carer. Communication is essential: talking about your feelings and limitations, expressing your needs.

It is also beneficial to seek support outside the family. Turning to support groups, therapists or specialist coaches can provide an outside perspective, tailored advice and a space to express frustrations and emotions.

Education and training can also play a preventive role. Understanding the disease, its stages, care and communication techniques, can help carers feel better equipped and less overwhelmed.

Finally, it's essential to remember that taking care of yourself is not a sign of selfishness. On the contrary, it's by being good to ourselves that we can be fully present for others. In the face of burnout, the key is to strike a balance between giving and receiving, between commitment and renewal.

The importance of supervision and peer support

Caring for people with Alzheimer's disease, with its specific challenges and emotional demands, highlights the vital importance of supervision and peer support. These two elements play a key role in the well-being of carers, whether professionals or family carers, and help to ensure quality care for patients.

Supervision, often provided by experienced professionals, offers a space for reflection, analysis and evaluation of practice. In the context of Alzheimer's, it gives carers the opportunity to examine their actions, emotional reactions and choices in the face of often complex situations. Supervision is an ideal opportunity to take a step back, acquire new skills and ensure that actions taken are in line with best practice in the field.

Peer support offers a complementary dimension. In these groups, carers can share their experiences, successes, challenges and concerns with others in similar situations. This professional or family solidarity helps to break the isolation that can sometimes be felt when faced with Alzheimer's disease. Peers can provide advice, strategies or simply an empathetic ear.

Beyond simple discussion, peer support is also a place of recognition. In the hustle and bustle of everyday life, seeing your efforts and dedication recognised by others is a powerful motivator. It's also a place where emotions, often bottled up in the context of work or care at home, can be expressed, heard and understood.

What's more, these exchanges often lead to the discovery of tips, techniques or resources that we didn't know existed. Peers, through their experience, are a mine of practical information and innovative approaches.

The importance of supervision and peer support cannot be underestimated. Both help to prevent professional and emotional burnout, ensure quality care and reinforce the sense of belonging to a community, whether professional or of family carers. In the often tortuous journey that is Alzheimer's care, supervision and peer support are like beacons of light, guiding and supporting carers every step of the way.

Relaxation techniques and stress management

Faced with the unique challenges of caring for patients with Alzheimer's disease, relaxation and stress management techniques are becoming essential tools for the well-being of carers. These techniques are not only beneficial for carers, but can also be adapted to help patients themselves manage their anxiety and tension.

- **Deep breathing:** The basis of many relaxation techniques. It consists of breathing in deeply through the nose, holding your breath for a few moments and then exhaling slowly through the mouth. This simple method rapidly reduces the heart rate and lowers blood pressure.

- **Meditation and mindfulness:** These techniques encourage people to focus their attention on the present moment. For carers, a few minutes' meditation a day can help reduce stress. For patients, mindfulness, adapted to their cognitive capacity, can help them connect with their immediate environment and reduce anxiety.

- **Visualisation exercises:** mentally projecting yourself into a soothing place, such as a beach or garden, can offer respite from the stresses of everyday life.

- **Muscle relaxation techniques:** These methods involve deliberately tensing and then relaxing different muscle groups in the body. They are particularly effective in relieving physical tension.

- **Yoga and tai chi:** These disciplines combine movement, breathing and meditation. They are excellent for strengthening the body, calming the mind and managing stress. What's more, adapted versions can be offered to patients, promoting their mobility and well-being.

- **Gratitude diary:** Taking a few moments each day to write down what you're grateful for can change your perspective on the challenges you face and boost your positive outlook.
- **Biofeedback techniques:** Using specialised equipment, these techniques teach you to voluntarily control certain physiological functions, such as heart rate, to manage stress.
- **Art and music therapy:** Expressing yourself through art or listening to soothing music are excellent ways for carers and patients to relax.
- **Outdoor activities:** Nature has a soothing effect. A simple walk, listening to birdsong or contemplating the landscape can be a source of deep relaxation.
- **Setting limits:** Knowing how to say 'no', delegating certain tasks and taking time for yourself are essential to prevent burnout.

It is essential for carers to remember that taking time for their own well-being is not a luxury, but a necessity. By taking care of themselves, they will be better equipped to provide the best possible care to their patients. Relaxation and stress management techniques are valuable tools in this ongoing effort to achieve balance and well-being.

Chapter 9:
CASE STUDIES: REAL-LIFE STORIES FROM ALZHEIMER'S UNITS

Resilience in the face of progress the disease

Alzheimer's disease is an ordeal, not only for the patients themselves, but also for the carers and families around them. The progression of the disease, with its increasing challenges and successive losses, requires remarkable inner strength to persevere. Resilience is the ability to face adversity, adapt and keep going despite the obstacles. It is an essential skill in the face of the progression of Alzheimer's disease.

The evolution of resilience :
- **Acknowledging reality**: Accepting the diagnosis and acknowledging the reality of the disease is the first step. This does not mean giving up hope, but rather understanding the situation so that you can deal with it proactively.
- **Seek support**: It's essential to surround yourself with a strong team, whether it's healthcare professionals, support groups, friends or family. Sharing emotions, challenges and successes builds resilience.
- **Finding meaning**: Understanding that, despite the illness, the person remains unique and valuable can help to find meaning in the process. This can also mean getting involved in raising awareness of the disease or in research.
- **Celebrating small victories**: As the disease progresses, it's crucial to celebrate every moment of

joy, every memory shared, every laugh. These moments become anchors that strengthen resilience.

- **Taking care of oneself**: Carers, in particular, need to look after their own well-being, both physical and emotional. This includes taking time for themselves, managing stress and finding fulfilling activities outside of care.
- **Education and information**: Understanding the disease, its symptoms and treatments can help you feel more in control. Education is a powerful tool for resilience.
- **Adaptability**: As the disease progresses, it's crucial to be flexible and adapt to new realities. This may mean rethinking routines, adapting the environment or revising expectations.
- **Maintaining a human connection**: Keeping in touch with the patient, even when communication becomes difficult, is essential. Affectionate gestures, music or simply being there can transcend the barriers of illness.

Resilience in the face of the progression of Alzheimer's disease is not a linear road, but rather a journey with its ups and downs. It is fuelled by love, determination, support and the ability to find light even in the darkest moments. Beyond the challenges, it is a testament to the incredible strength of the human spirit.

Navigate through
the complexities of communication

Navigating the complexities of communication with an Alzheimer's patient requires both patience and a tailored approach. The disease, with its degenerative effects on cognitive abilities, can make communication difficult, but not impossible. Understanding these complexities is essential to maintaining a human connection with the patient throughout the progression of the disease.

The challenges of communicating with Alzheimer's disease :

- **Language disturbance**: Patients may have difficulty finding the right words, forming complete sentences or following a conversation.
- **Memory problems**: Frequent forgetfulness, difficulty recognising familiar faces or remembering recent events can hamper communication.
- **Perceptual difficulties**: Problems such as misinterpretation of non-verbal cues or increased sensitivity to noise can disrupt communication.

Strategies for effective communication :
- **Simplicity and clarity**: Use short sentences, simple words and speak slowly. Make sure your message is understood before moving on to the next one.
- **Keep a positive tone**: A warm tone, a patient attitude and eye contact can make communication more accessible.
- **Avoid distractions**: Minimise background noise, turn off the television and make sure you have the patient's attention before you speak.
- **Use non-verbal language**: Gestures, facial expressions and touch can convey as much or more than words.
- **Validate and comfort**: If the patient is confused or anxious, it's often better to validate their feelings rather than correct them.
- **Use visual aids**: Photos, objects or memory aids can make communication easier.
- **Repeat or rephrase if necessary**: If the patient doesn't understand, try rephrasing rather than repeating exactly the same sentence.

- **Encourage simple choices**: Rather than asking an open-ended question, offer two choices to make the decision easier.
- **Listen with patience**: Even if the speech is disorganised, the act of listening is a gesture of respect and compassion.

Anticipating and adapting to change :
As the illness progresses, communication can become increasingly difficult. It is crucial to be flexible, to adapt methods and to accept that, sometimes, simple presence and physical contact can be the most powerful forms of communication.

Navigating the complexities of communication in the context of Alzheimer's disease is as much an art as a science. It is a journey of continuous learning, with each patient offering a unique lesson in the nature of human connection and the importance of patience, understanding and love.

Love and compassion
at the heart of care

Love and compassion are much more than just emotions or gestures. In the context of caring for people with Alzheimer's disease, these two elements become the cornerstone of a therapeutic approach that goes beyond medication or clinical interventions. They are the very substance that weaves the bond between caregiver and patient, offering a glimmer of humanity in a landscape often darkened by the disease.

Love as a foundation :
Beyond its traditional definition, love in this context is a profound appreciation of the other person's humanity, a

recognition of their intrinsic value. Alzheimer's patients, despite the loss of certain abilities, remain human beings with desires, memories and a history. Loving these patients means recognising their individuality and dignity, even when they can no longer do so themselves.

Compassion as a method of care :
Compassion is an empathetic response to the suffering of others. It requires the carer to put themselves in the patient's shoes, to feel what they are feeling, and to act accordingly. In moments of confusion or distress, an act of compassion can soothe, reassure and comfort.

Tangible benefits:
- **Reduced anxiety**: A loving, compassionate approach reassures patients and reduces the anxiety often associated with illness.
- **Cognitive stimulation**: A warm, loving environment can have a positive effect on cognition, encouraging moments of clarity and connection.
- **Improved physical care**: A caring approach makes medical procedures and daily routines easier to manage for the patient.

For carers:
Compassion and love are just as beneficial for the carer. They give deep meaning to the work they do, strengthen bonds and provide a source of energy at otherwise exhausting times.
However, making such an emotionally intense commitment is not without its challenges. There can be a high risk of burnout, sadness at the progression of the disease or difficulty in managing emotions.
The need for balance :

It is crucial for carers to find a balance. This means allowing themselves breaks, seeking support, and recognising their own emotions and needs. Compassion for oneself is just as important as compassion for patients.

Love and compassion, when integrated into the heart of Alzheimer's care, can transform the experience of the disease for everyone involved. They are a reminder that, beyond the symptoms, medications and challenges, there is an individual who deserves respect, dignity and affection. In this sacred space of care, even in the midst of decline and loss, moments of beauty, joy and humanity can still flourish.

Chapter 10:
ETHICAL AND LEGAL ASPECTS

The rights of Alzheimer's patients

The rights of Alzheimer's patients are of crucial importance. These individuals, although facing cognitive deterioration, have the same fundamental rights as any other person. However, due to the progressive and debilitating nature of their disease, they may require a more vigorous defence of their rights.

Recognition of individuality :
Each Alzheimer's patient is first and foremost an individual, with his or her own history, values, wishes and needs. Despite the disease, their individuality must always be respected and recognised.

The right to dignified and respectful care:
- **Quality care**: Alzheimer's patients have the right to receive care that is adapted to their needs, respects their preferences and is provided by trained and competent professionals.
- **Protection against abuse**: Like any vulnerable person, they have the right to be protected against any form of abuse, whether physical, emotional, financial or other.

Participation in decision-making :
Even with reduced cognitive capacity, patients have the right to be informed and, as far as possible, to participate in decision-making about their care, treatment and daily life.

Right to privacy and confidentiality :
The privacy of Alzheimer's patients must be respected, whether in terms of their medical data, their physical intimacy or their personal communications.

Access to appropriate therapies and treatments :
This includes not only medical treatments, but also non-pharmacological interventions such as art and music therapies and cognitive stimulation.

The right to live in a safe and stimulating environment :
Alzheimer's patients have the right to live in a safe environment, where the risks of falls, wandering off or other dangers are minimised, while benefiting from stimulating activities adapted to their abilities.

Right to information :
Patients and their families have the right to be informed about the disease, its progression, treatment options and available resources.

Recognition of and respect for advance directives :
If a patient has drawn up advance directives or appointed a proxy in the event of incapacity, these choices must be respected and applied.

Right to non-discrimination :
Alzheimer's disease, although it has an impact on cognition, should not be a reason for treating these patients unequally or stigmatising them.

The rights of Alzheimer's patients reflect a person-centred approach that aims to ensure their well-being and to treat them with dignity and respect. While recognising the challenges posed by the disease, it is essential for carers, families and society in general to defend these rights vigorously, ensuring that every Alzheimer's patient is treated with the humanity and consideration they deserve.

Medical decision-making and informed consent

Medical decision-making and informed consent are central to modern medicine, emphasising respect for individual autonomy and the need for open communication between patient and healthcare professional. However, when it comes to patients with Alzheimer's disease, these concepts take on a particularly complex dimension.

Principle of informed consent :
Informed consent is based on the idea that an individual has the right to make decisions about his or her own body and health. Before any medical intervention or procedure, the patient must be properly informed of the risks, benefits, possible alternatives and potential consequences. Only after receiving and understanding this information can the patient give informed consent.

Challenges posed by Alzheimer's disease :
- **Reduced cognitive capacity**: Alzheimer's patients may have difficulty understanding complex information, weighing up the pros and cons or expressing their preferences clearly.
- **Variability in decision-making ability**: The ability to make decisions may vary according to the stage of the disease, the time of day, or other factors.

Approaches to medical decision-making :
- **Assessment of decision-making capacity**: Before seeking consent, it is crucial to assess the patient's capacity to understand and make decisions.

Specialised tools and assessments are available for this purpose.

- **Involving family and friends**: If a patient is unable to give informed consent, it may be necessary to involve family and friends or a designated proxy to help in the decision-making process.
- **Advance directives**: These documents, drawn up when the patient is still fully capable, express the patient's wishes regarding medical care, interventions and treatment in the event of future incapacity to make decisions.
- **Simplified communication**: To facilitate understanding, it can be useful to adapt language, use visual aids or other means to present information clearly and concisely.

The role of healthcare professionals :
It is crucial for healthcare professionals to respect patients' autonomy while ensuring their safety and well-being. This may require delicate discussions, careful listening and attention to non-verbal cues.

Medical decision-making and informed consent for Alzheimer's patients are complex processes that require sensitivity, patience and skill. Although the disease can impair decision-making capacity, the importance of respecting the patient's dignity, rights and wishes remains paramount. A person-centred approach, combined with close collaboration with families and carers, can provide a balanced and ethical way of navigating these delicate waters.

Management of cases of abuse and negligence

Managing cases of abuse and neglect of people with Alzheimer's disease is a delicate, urgent and essential task. Because of their heightened vulnerability, these individuals are often at risk of exploitation, abuse or neglect. Dealing with this subject requires a combination of sensitivity, professional competence and moral commitment.

Types of abuse encountered :
- **Physical abuse:** Acts of violence or rough treatment.
- **Emotional abuse**: Insults, humiliation, threats or isolation.
- **Sexual abuse:** Any non-consensual sexual act.
- **Financial abuse**: Financial exploitation, theft or misappropriation of funds.
- **Neglect**: Failure to provide basic care, such as feeding, hygiene or taking medication.

Recognising the signs :
Healthcare professionals, particularly those working in Alzheimer's units, need to be trained to recognise subtle signs of abuse or neglect. These may include unexplained behavioural changes, recurrent injuries, signs of emotional distress or isolation, financial abnormalities, or declining health for no apparent medical reason.

Intervention protocols :
- **Accurate documentation:** It is essential to document any suspicious signs or symptoms in detail, including detailed descriptions, photos if necessary, and any other relevant information.

- **Confidentiality**: Protecting patient privacy is paramount, except in cases of immediate risk.
- **Reporting**: In the event of justified suspicion of abuse or negligence, a report must be made to the competent authorities.
- **Patient support**: Providing a safe environment and offering psychological and medical support tailored to the patient.

Prevention :
- **Staff training**: All healthcare professionals should receive specific training in the recognition and management of abuse and neglect.
- **Regular assessments**: Regular assessments of the patient's physical and emotional well-being can help detect and prevent abuse.
- **Open communication**: Encouraging open communication between staff, patients and families can help prevent or detect abuse.
- **Clear protocols**: Having standardised procedures for dealing with allegations of abuse ensures that cases are dealt with quickly and effectively.

Managing cases of abuse and neglect of Alzheimer's patients is a grave responsibility for all healthcare professionals. Over and above professional skills, it requires genuine humanity, constant vigilance and an unwavering commitment to the protection and well-being of these particularly vulnerable individuals. Every case of abuse or neglect is a tragedy, but with the right training, awareness and effective action protocols, these events can be minimised or even eliminated.

Chapter 11:
NUTRITION AND FOOD CARE

Nutritional challenges
in Alzheimer's patients

Nutrition plays a crucial role in the general well-being of every individual. For people with Alzheimer's disease, maintaining a balanced diet can present unique challenges. Cognitive, behavioural and physiological changes associated with the disease can interfere with adequate dietary intake, and recognising and managing these challenges is essential to supporting the patient's health and quality of life.

Changes in perception and preferences :
As the disease progresses, patients may lose their taste for certain foods or develop sudden aversions. These changes may be due to alterations in the perception of taste and smell. Food preferences may also be influenced by psychological or emotional factors, such as anxiety or depression.

Problems with chewing and swallowing :
Patients may have difficulty chewing or swallowing certain foods, increasing the risk of choking or malnutrition. This may be due to a loss of muscle coordination or to changes in the structure of the mouth.

Reduced appetite :
Some Alzheimer's patients may lose their appetite, either as a result of the disease itself or because of prescribed medication. This can lead to unwanted weight loss and nutritional deficiencies.

Forgetting to eat:
The memory loss common in Alzheimer's patients can lead them to forget to eat or to eat several times thinking they haven't done so.

Behavioural difficulties :
Behaviours such as agitation, confusion or distractibility can make eating difficult. In addition, some patients may have fixations or compulsions around certain foods.

Coping strategies :
- **Soothing meal environment**: Creating a calm, distraction-free environment can help focus the patient's attention on the meal.
- **Familiar and favourite foods**: Serving foods that the patient recognises and enjoys can encourage food intake.
- **Assistance with meals**: Some patients may need help with eating, whether it's cutting up food or being guided through a meal.
- **Nutritional supplements**: If food intake is insufficient, nutritional supplements may be considered to ensure adequate intake.
- **Regular monitoring of weight and nutrition**: Regular monitoring of weight, food intake and levels of essential nutrients can help to identify any potential problems early on.
- **Alternative therapies**: Music therapy or aromatherapy can stimulate the appetite or create an atmosphere more conducive to eating.

Dealing with the nutritional challenges of Alzheimer's patients requires a holistic approach that takes into account both the medical and psychosocial aspects of the disease. Through careful observation, flexibility and close collaboration with dieticians, carers and families, it is possible to overcome these obstacles and ensure optimal nutrition for patients throughout their journey with Alzheimer's disease.

Techniques to encourage eating and hydration

Encouraging nutrition and hydration in Alzheimer's patients is essential to maintain their physical health, prevent medical complications and support their general well-being. Here are some techniques for achieving this smoothly and effectively:

1. Creating the right environment :
   - **Calm atmosphere**: Reduce distractions such as television or radio during meals to help the patient concentrate on eating.
   - **Attractive set-up**: Present the food in an appetising way, with varied colours and well-arranged plates. Contrasting plates can help patients to see the food more clearly.
2. Adapting food preferences :
   - **Familiar food**: Familiar dishes can arouse the patient's interest in food, evoking pleasant memories.
   - **Varied textures**: If chewing or swallowing becomes a problem, try softer or puréed foods. Smoothies and soups can also be good options.
3. To be present at meals:
   - **Eating together**: The simple act of sharing a meal can encourage a patient to eat.
   - **Manual guidance**: For more advanced patients, gently guiding their hand to help them eat may be necessary.

4. Split meals :
   - **Frequent small meals**: Instead of three big meals, try giving smaller portions more frequently throughout the day.
5. Hydration :
   - **Regular reminders**: Encourage patients to drink regularly, even if they don't feel thirsty.
   - **A variety of drinks**: teas, juices, soups, flavoured water or smoothies can make hydration more appealing.
   - **Spot the signs of dehydration**: Dry skin, confusion or dark urine can be signs of insufficient hydration.
6. Reinforcement techniques :
   - **Praise and encouragement**: Praise the patient's efforts, even if they are minimal.
   - **Involve the patient**: Involve him or her in preparing meals or choosing food, which may arouse their interest in food.
7. Use of appropriate tools :
   - **Ergonomic utensils**: Adapted cutlery or cups with large handles can make eating easier.
   - **Check the temperature**: Make sure the food and drinks are neither too hot nor too cold.

8. Pay attention to nutritional requirements :
   - **Supplements**: If food intake is insufficient, discuss with a nutritionist the possibility of introducing supplements to guarantee nutritional requirements.
   - **Detecting deficiencies**: Regular check-ups can help identify any early nutritional deficiencies.

Nutrition and hydration are fundamental elements in the care of Alzheimer's patients. Approaching them with patience, creativity and compassion can make all the difference to the patient's well-being. By being attentive to the unique needs of the patient, adapting techniques and collaborating with healthcare professionals, carers can overcome nutritional challenges and ensure optimal care.

Managing swallowing disorders and aspirations

Dysphagia, or difficulty swallowing, is a common condition in people with Alzheimer's disease and other forms of dementia. Proper management of these problems is essential to prevent complications such as malnutrition, dehydration, and particularly aspiration, which can lead to pneumonia.

Recognising symptoms:
- **Coughing or choking** on food or drink.
- **Change in voice** after drinking or eating (wet or slurred voice).
- **Retention of food in** the mouth or difficulty starting to swallow.
- Unexplained **weight loss** and reduced appetite.

Strategies for managing dysphagia:
- **Professional consultation**: It is important to have an assessment by a speech and language therapist, who can offer specific advice on managing dysphagia.
- Change in consistency of food :
    - Pureed or chopped food to make swallowing easier.
    - Use thickeners for liquids if necessary.
- Appropriate   position during and after meals:
    - Make sure the patient is sitting upright at a 90-degree angle during meals.
    - Avoid putting the patient to bed immediately after eating or drinking.

- Swallowing techniques :
    - Encourage multiple swallowing to ensure that all the food has gone down.
    - Use techniques such as chin-tuck swallowing (head tilted downwards) to help protect the airways.
- **Careful monitoring**: Watch out for signs of aspiration, such as coughing, changes in skin colour or wheezing.
- **Maintaining good oral hygiene**: Food remains in the mouth can be aspirated later, so it's essential to make sure the mouth is clean after meals.

Aspiration prevention:
- **Regular monitoring**: Regularly check the patient's lung condition, listen to breathing.
- **Avoid distractions**: Meals should take place in a calm environment to allow the patient to concentrate on swallowing.
- **Take frequent breaks**: Let the patient catch their breath between mouthfuls or sips.
- **Consult regularly**: Regular assessments by professionals can help identify and correct problems before they become serious.

Dysphagia and the risk of aspiration are serious challenges for people with Alzheimer's disease. Proactive and informed management can prevent serious complications. With the right training, constant vigilance and professional support, carers can provide safe and effective care for their patients while allowing them to enjoy their meals.

Chapter 12:
MOBILISATION AND FALLS PREVENTION

Understanding the risks of falls in Alzheimer's patients

Falls are a major concern for the elderly, and even more so for people with Alzheimer's disease. Cognitive decline, sensory and motor changes, as well as medication, can increase the risk of falls in these patients. Understanding and minimising these risks is essential to ensure patient safety.

Risk factors :
- **Problems with walking and balance**: As the disease progresses, the patient's motor functions may deteriorate, making it difficult to walk and maintain balance.
- **Visual deterioration**: Visual perception may be affected, making it difficult to distinguish obstacles, edges or changes in ground levels.
- **Confusion and disorientation**: Patients may not recognise their surroundings, try to get up at night or have hallucinations that cause them to move suddenly.
- **Side effects of medication**: Some medicines, particularly those for anxiety, depression or sleep disorders, can cause dizziness or a drop in blood pressure.
- **Environmental obstacles**: Poorly placed furniture, electrical wires, carpets and lack of lighting can all contribute to falls.

Prevention strategies :
- **Regular assessment:** It is crucial to regularly assess the patient's motor skills, as well as their environment, to identify potential risks.
- Home security :
  - Remove obstacles from the ground.
  - Install grab rails in the bathroom and by the bed.
  - Use non-slip mats.
  - Ensure adequate lighting, particularly at night.
  - Opt for suitable   footwear with good support and non-slip soles.
- **Regular   exercise**: Encourage patients to do gentle exercises such as walking or tai chi, which can improve balance and muscle strength.
- **Medication review**: Work with a doctor to ensure that prescribed medication does not unnecessarily increase the risk of falling.
- **Training and awareness**: Train carers and family members to recognise the risks of falls and to intervene accordingly.

Falls among Alzheimer's patients are not inevitable. By understanding the associated risks and implementing preventive measures, the number of incidents can be greatly reduced. It's a process that requires constant attention, ongoing assessment and close collaboration between carers, health professionals and the family to ensure patient safety.

Appropriate mobilisation techniques

Mobilising Alzheimer's patients requires special attention, not only because of the physical challenges, but also because of the cognitive ones. The disease can impair the patient's perception, ability to follow instructions and motor coordination. Mobilisation techniques must therefore be adapted to ensure the patient's safety and comfort, while respecting their dignity.

General principles of mobilisation :
- **Communication**: Before any mobilisation, speak gently and clearly to the patient, explaining what you are going to do.
- **Calm approach**: Sudden or unexpected movements can cause anxiety or resistance.
- **Safety first**: Make sure the environment is safe, with non-slip surfaces and no obstacles.

Specific techniques :
- Bed-to-chair transfer :
  - Use sliding sheets or transfer boards if necessary.
  - Make sure the patient is sitting on the edge of the bed with their feet firmly on the floor before getting up.
  - Offer support under the arms and make sure they are able to bear their weight before moving them completely.
- Walking :
  - If the patient is unstable, use a walking belt or a walker.
  - Walk beside them, slightly backwards, ready to provide support.
  - Encourage slow, steady   steps, avoiding uneven surfaces.
- Passive mobilisation :
  - When the patient is bedridden and unable to move around on their own, perform passive movements to avoid stiff joints.
  - Gently support the limb and move it through its normal range of movement.

Use of assistive devices :

Mechanical   patient lifts can be used for patients who are unable to bear their own weight.

Make sure that the straps are secure and that the patient is comfortable during the process.

Hygiene and personal care :

When helping the patient with their personal care, make sure they are well supported. For example, when bathing, use a shower chair with non-slip   feet.

Points to consider:

Pain can affect the ability to mobilise. Make sure the patient is comfortable and consider painkillers if necessary.

Regularly assess the patient's ability to mobilise and adapt techniques accordingly.

Involve the patient as much as possible, and encourage them to help as much as they can.

Ensure that all staff are trained in appropriate mobilisation techniques.

Mobilising Alzheimer's patients can be challenging, but with the right approach, it can be done safely and effectively. It is an essential component of care for these patients, helping to prevent complications such as pressure sores and loss of muscle strength, while promoting general well-being.

Safety features and equipment

When working with Alzheimer's patients, safety is an absolute priority. These patients can exhibit unpredictable behaviour, reduced perception of danger and impaired sense of direction. So creating a safe, appropriate environment is essential to prevent accidents and promote a sense of well-being.

General fittings :

- **Lighting**: Good lighting is crucial to preventing falls. Use motion-detecting lights to automatically illuminate areas when a person approaches, such as corridors and bathrooms.
- **Floors**: Avoid carpets, which can create obstacles. Opt for non-slip floor coverings, particularly in bathrooms.
- **Clear signage**: Signs with images can help patients find their way around and identify rooms, such as toilets or their own bedroom.
- **Grab bars**: Install them in bathrooms, toilets and near the bed to help with mobilisation.
- **Surveillance cameras**: In some cases, to ensure the safety of high-risk patients, cameras can be installed to monitor movements and prevent incidents.

Specific safety devices :

- **Motion detectors**: These devices can alert staff if a patient leaves their bed or room during the night.
- **Identification wristbands**: These can be fitted with GPS chips to locate patients who might get lost.
- **Secure doors**: Access codes or badge systems can prevent patients from leaving unsupervised.
- **Fall risk reducers**: These include low beds, floor mats placed next to the bed, and non-slip footwear.
- **Alert systems**: Call buttons or portable devices allow patients to signal if they need help.
- **Rounded corners on furniture**: This can prevent injury in the event of a fall.

Special zones :

Secure gardens: A fenced-in, supervised outdoor area allows patients to enjoy the outdoors in complete safety.

Relaxation areas: Calm, soothing rooms can help manage patients' agitation or anxiety.

Education and training :

In addition to physical accommodation, staff should be trained in fall prevention techniques, managing difficult behaviour and responding to emergencies. Regular simulations and reminders of safety procedures can help to ensure that patients are protected.

Creating a safe environment for Alzheimer's patients goes beyond simply preventing accidents. It helps to create an atmosphere in which patients feel safe, respected and cared for. By implementing these features and safety devices, it is possible to offer high-quality care while minimising risks.

Chapter 13:
DEATH AND PALLIATIVE CARE

A sensitive approach to the end of life

The care of patients with advanced Alzheimer's disease and the approach of the end of life are delicate periods that require particular attention and sensitivity. This involves not only ensuring that the patient receives appropriate medical care, but also ensuring that his or her emotional, psychological and spiritual needs are taken into account. Approaching the end of life with sensitivity requires compassion, empathy and open communication with the patient, family and care team.

1. Recognising the signs of the end of life :
Alzheimer's patients may present symptoms such as cognitive deterioration, loss of appetite, increasing immobility, frequent infections or a general deterioration in health. Recognising these signs means that care can be better prepared and adapted.

2. Communication with the family :
Engage in open and honest conversations with the family about the course of the illness, palliative care options and the patient's end-of-life wishes. Be sure to choose an appropriate time, in a calm setting, for these sensitive discussions.

3. Palliative care :
The aim is to relieve pain and other uncomfortable symptoms, while supporting the patient's emotional and spiritual needs. The emphasis is on quality of life rather than length of life.

4. Respecting the patient's wishes :
If the patient has drawn up advance directives or a power of attorney for healthcare, it is imperative that their wishes regarding medical treatment, intervention and the end of life are respected.

5. Emotional support :
Offer regular psychological support sessions or music and art therapies to help patients express their emotions and find a sense of calm.

6. Spirituality :
If the patient is religious or spiritual, incorporate practices or rituals that are important to them, such as prayer, meditation or specific rituals.

7. Preparing for the aftermath :
Guide the family through the grieving process, helping them to anticipate and understand the emotions they may be feeling. Offer resources such as support groups or bereavement counsellors.

8. Farewell rituals :
Allow the family to spend time with the patient, talking to them, holding their hand or listening to their favourite music. These moments can help bring closure.

Approaching the end of life for Alzheimer's patients with sensitivity is a complex process that encompasses not only the medical aspects, but also emotions, spirituality and human dignity. It is a time when compassion, respect and empathy take on their full meaning. As a healthcare professional, it is essential to gently guide the patient and their family through this stage, ensuring that all their needs are respected and supported.

Palliative care
specific to Alzheimer's patients

Palliative care plays a vital role in supporting Alzheimer's patients, particularly in the advanced stages of the disease. This care is not limited to simply managing physical pain, but also encompasses the psychological, social and spiritual aspects of well-being. It aims to improve the patient's quality of life and support their family. For Alzheimer's patients, palliative care takes on special characteristics that reflect the complexity of the disease.

1. Overall assessment of needs :
Regular assessment of the patient's needs is fundamental to adapting care to the progression of the disease. This includes assessing pain (which is often underestimated or misinterpreted in these patients), behavioural symptoms and nutritional needs.

2. Pain management :
Impaired communication makes it difficult for patients to express their pain. It is therefore crucial to use appropriate pain measurement scales and to remain attentive to non-verbal signs such as agitation, refusal to eat or withdrawal.

3. Non-pharmacological approach :
In addition to medication, complementary therapies such as music therapy, art therapy or massage therapy can help to ease symptoms and provide comfort.

4. Management of neuropsychiatric symptoms :
Patients may experience symptoms such as agitation, aggression or depression. A combination of medicinal and non-medicinal approaches is often required to manage them.

5. Nutritional support :
As the disease progresses, problems with feeding may arise. Regular assessment of nutritional status, the use of appropriate foods or enteral feeding may be considered.

6. Appropriate communication :
The communication approach must be modified to meet the needs of patients who may have difficulty understanding or expressing themselves. Simple, clear and repetitive communication is preferable.

7. Emotional and spiritual support :
Respecting the patient's beliefs and values is essential. The use of chaplains, counsellors or other spiritual professionals can offer valuable support.

8. Support for families :
Families often need guidance, education and emotional support. Helping them understand what to expect, providing resources and supporting them in their grieving process are all essential.

9. Advance care planning :
Although difficult, it is important to discuss the patient's wishes regarding care with the family, particularly on issues such as resuscitation, artificial nutrition and hospitalisation.

10. Place of care :
The decision as to where care will be provided (at home, in a hospice, in a specialist unit) must be based on the patient's needs, the family's wishes and the resources available.

Palliative care for Alzheimer's patients requires a holistic, individualised and patient-centred approach. It requires close collaboration between different healthcare professionals to ensure optimal care for both the patient and his or her family.

Supporting families through bereavement

Alzheimer's disease is an ordeal that often lasts for many years, and throughout this period, families experience successive bereavements, ranging from the gradual loss of their loved one's cognitive abilities to their physical demise. Bereavement support is an essential aspect of care, enabling families to find a degree of peace and to rebuild their lives after the loss.

1. Anticipated mourning:
Even before the patient's death, families experience what is known as "anticipated mourning". They mourn the loss of their loved one's memories, personality and abilities. It's a complex process, because it's mixed with the pain of seeing the loved one move away, while still being physically present.

2. Recognising the uniqueness of bereavement:
Every family and every individual experiences bereavement differently. It is essential to recognise this uniqueness, not to judge, and to provide support tailored to each situation.

3. Providing information:
Understanding the disease process, its stages and the emotional reactions it generates can help families to manage their grief more effectively. Information sessions and open discussions can be organised on a regular basis.

4. Offer psychological support:
Individual or group therapy sessions, led by trained professionals, can help families to express their feelings, manage their pain and find strategies for moving forward.

5. Encourage support groups:
Support groups provide a place for families to share their experiences, difficulties and coping strategies. These meetings reinforce the feeling that they are not alone in the face of illness.

6. Organising rituals:
Rituals, whether religious or not, can help give meaning to the loss, celebrate the life of the deceased and begin the healing process.

7. Encourage the expression of feelings:
It is important to allow families to express their feelings, whether sad, angry, guilty or otherwise. Expression can take many forms: discussion, writing, art, music, etc.

8. Prepare for the post-mourning phase:
It is crucial to support families in the aftermath, by helping them to envisage life without their loved one, to regain their balance and to plan new projects or activities.

Supporting families in their bereavement is a delicate journey that requires listening, compassion and expertise. It is a process that is not limited to the immediate aftermath of the death, but is a long-term one. Acknowledging the depth of their grief and offering appropriate support helps to ease the burden on families and guide them towards healing.

Chapter 14:
TECHNOLOGICAL TOOLS
IN ALZHEIMER'S UNITS

The use of technology
to improve care

In an era dominated by technological developments, it is only natural to integrate these innovations into the world of care, and particularly into the treatment and care of patients suffering from Alzheimer's disease. Far from being mere gadgets, these technologies can bring about significant changes, not only in the lives of patients, but also in those of healthcare professionals and their families.

1. Assistance and monitoring technologies:
Devices such as GPS watches can help track patients' movements, minimising the risk of them wandering off. In addition, motion sensors and cameras can be installed in homes or care facilities to monitor patients' activities, ensuring their safety.

2. Improved communication:
Specific applications have been designed to facilitate communication between patients and their relatives or carers. These visual and auditory tools can help overcome the language and cognitive barriers that arise as the disease progresses.

3. Virtual reality:
Virtual reality has shown promise in helping patients to relive memories, visit familiar places or take part in therapeutic activities, thereby contributing to their emotional and cognitive well-being.

4. Cognitive stimulation games and applications:
Many interactive games have been developed for tablets and computers, targeting memory, attention and other cognitive functions. These games can be both entertaining and beneficial for maintaining mental capacity.

5. Telemedicine and remote monitoring:
Telemedicine enables doctors and healthcare professionals to monitor patients remotely, providing access to care without the need for frequent travel, which can be particularly useful for patients living in remote areas.

6. Robotics and artificial intelligence:
AI-equipped robots have been introduced in some establishments to help with patient care, whether for monitoring, social interaction or even tasks such as dispensing medication.

7. Databases and electronic medical records:
The use of electronic medical records enables better coordination between different healthcare professionals, guaranteeing more coherent and efficient care.

The integration of technology into the care of Alzheimer's patients is opening up new doors, both in terms of efficiency of care and quality of life for patients. However, it is essential to ensure that these innovations are used judiciously, complementing traditional approaches and always in the best interests of the patient.

Surveillance and security tools

When caring for patients with Alzheimer's disease, safety is a major concern. As the disease progresses, patients can be prone to unpredictable behaviour, disorientation and even running away. Modern technology offers a range of tools which, if used properly, can ensure greater safety for these patients while preserving their dignity.

1. Geolocation devices:
   - **GPS watches**: These discreet, easy-to-wear watches track the patient's position in real time. They can also be programmed to send alerts if the patient leaves a defined area.
   - **GPS insoles**: For patients who would otherwise be able to remove a watch, GPS-equipped insoles can be placed in their shoes.
2. Alarms and motion sensors:
   - **Door sensors**: These emit an alert if a door is open, particularly useful for preventing people from going out at night.
   - **Motion detectors**: These can be used to monitor specific areas, such as the entrance to a house or a room.
3. Surveillance cameras:
   - Strategically placed, they enable carers to monitor certain rooms remotely, guaranteeing patient safety while offering a degree of autonomy.
   - Mobile applications are often available for real-time monitoring.
4. Communication devices:
   - **Intercoms**: Enable communication between different rooms, ideal for reassuring a patient or intervening quickly.
   - **Communicating watches**: In addition to geolocation, some watches enable direct communication with the wearer.
5. Medical alert systems:
   - **Emergency buttons**: Worn around the neck or on the wrist, these buttons, when activated, send an alert to a control centre or to a relative.

6. Dedicated mobile applications:
   There are a number of apps specifically designed to help carers monitor Alzheimer's patients, including functions such as medication reminders, geolocation and direct communication.
7. Drug blocking and home security devices:
   Lockable medicine boxes prevent accidental overdoses.
   Protectors for hobs or other dangerous household appliances prevent accidents in the home.

While exploiting the benefits of these monitoring and safety tools, it is essential to respect the patient's privacy and dignity. The use of these devices must be done with consent and transparency, ensuring that the patient and their family are informed and comfortable with the measures put in place.

Technology as a means communication and commitment

Technological developments have transformed the way we communicate and interact. For Alzheimer's patients, these innovations can offer new ways of communicating, as well as revitalising their engagement with the world around them, despite the obstacles posed by the disease.

1. Tablets and specific applications:
Tablets, with their intuitive interface, are invaluable tools. Dedicated applications allow patients to take part in memory games, express their emotions, or simply communicate with their loved ones via video calls.

2. Virtual and augmented reality:
These immersive technologies can be used to take patients back to familiar environments, help them relive memories

or even for relaxation therapies. They offer a multi-sensory experience that can be tailored to the patient's specific needs.

3. Music and video platforms:
Music has the power to trigger memories and emotions. Thanks to platforms such as Spotify and YouTube, it is possible to create personalised playlists that remind patients of precious moments in their lives.

4. Adapted video games:
Some video games have been specially designed for people with dementia, stimulating their cognition while providing them with moments of fun.
5. Social robots:
Robots such as Paro, the interactive seal, and Pepper have been designed to interact socially with patients, providing them with a source of companionship and interaction.

6. Communicating watches and wristbands:
In addition to simple monitoring, some of these devices enable two-way interaction, allowing the patient to convey a message or express a need.

7. Online forums and communities:
For family and friends, these spaces offer an opportunity to share, learn and find support. Sometimes patients themselves, especially in the early stages of the disease, can benefit from these exchanges.

By breaking down traditional communication barriers, technology is opening up promising avenues for engaging with Alzheimer's patients. However, it is essential to adapt these tools to the individual needs of each patient and to integrate them into a holistic approach to care. Always at the forefront, we must also ensure that these technological innovations are accessible to all, so that every patient can benefit from advances in this field.

Chapter 15:
RESEARCH AND ITS IMPACT
ON NURSING PRACTICE

Current advances in Alzheimer's research

Alzheimer's disease is complex and multifactorial, and is the subject of intense research worldwide. In recent years, major advances have been made in elucidating certain mechanisms of the disease and opening up new therapeutic avenues. Here is an overview of the main advances and trends in current Alzheimer's research.

1. Identification of biomarkers:
Advances in medical imaging and molecular biology have enabled the identification of specific biomarkers, such as the Tau and beta-amyloid proteins, present in abnormal quantities in patients' brains. These biomarkers offer new tools for early diagnosis and monitoring of the disease.

2. Gene therapies:
Specific genetic mutations are associated with an increased risk of developing Alzheimer's disease. Gene therapy aims to correct or replace these defective genes, offering an innovative approach to treatment.

3. Role of the intestinal microbiota:
Recent studies suggest a link between the intestinal microbiota and the development of Alzheimer's disease. Interactions between certain types of intestinal bacteria and the brain could play a role in the pathogenesis of the disease.

4. Vaccines and immunotherapies:
There are initiatives to develop vaccines targeting the abnormal proteins associated with Alzheimer's. Immunotherapy aims to use the body's immune system to fight or prevent the disease.

5. Neuroplasticity and neurogenesis:
Research has highlighted the brain's potential to regenerate and create new connections. Stimulating this capacity could be a promising way of slowing or reversing Alzheimer's symptoms.

6. The role of inflammation:
Chronic inflammation of the brain is now recognised as a key factor in the progression of the disease. Anti-inflammatory drugs are therefore being studied as potential treatments.

7. Non-drug therapies:
In addition to drugs, the impact of diet, physical exercise and psychosocial interventions is increasingly being studied for their potential to prevent or slow the progression of the disease.

Although Alzheimer's disease remains a major challenge for medical research, recent advances offer a glimmer of hope. The current multidisciplinary approach, combining genetics, biology, neuroscience and even microbiology, suggests that more effective solutions for preventing, diagnosing and treating Alzheimer's may soon be available.

How research influences clinical management

Constantly evolving medical research plays a fundamental role in the way diseases are understood, diagnosed and treated. In the case of Alzheimer's disease, advances in research have directly influenced clinical management. Here is an exploration of the symbiosis between research and the clinic.

1. Early diagnosis:
Advances in biomarker research and medical imaging have enabled earlier and more accurate diagnosis of Alzheimer's disease. This means that patients can benefit from treatment and support more quickly, potentially slowing the progression of the disease.

2. Targeted treatments:
In-depth research into the molecular and genetic mechanisms of the disease has led to the development of specifically targeted drugs and therapeutic approaches. Although some of these treatments are still undergoing evaluation, they promise greater efficacy with fewer side effects.

3. Customised approaches:
The era of personalised medicine is upon us. Understanding genetic variability and individual profiles can guide clinicians towards tailor-made treatments that optimise outcomes for each patient.

4. Non-drug interventions:
Research into non-pharmacological interventions, such as cognitive stimulation and music therapy, has proven their effectiveness. Such methods are now routinely incorporated into care plans, offering a holistic approach to treatment.

5. Prevention and awareness-raising:
Epidemiological studies and research into risk factors have contributed to a better understanding of preventive measures. Clinicians are now better equipped to advise

patients and their families on lifestyle modifications that can reduce the risk of developing the disease.

6. Interdisciplinary collaboration:
The complexity of Alzheimer's requires an interdisciplinary approach. Research has highlighted the importance of collaboration between neurologists, psychologists, physiotherapists, occupational therapists and other specialists in providing comprehensive care.

7. Training and education of professionals:
Research findings are incorporated into training programmes for healthcare professionals, ensuring that patient care is at the cutting edge of current knowledge.

Research into Alzheimer's disease is a key driver in the continuous improvement of clinical care. Each new discovery, whether it concerns fundamental biology or therapeutic interventions, enriches the range of tools available to clinicians to provide the best possible care for patients. In turn, clinical observations often inspire new avenues of research, creating a virtuous circle of innovation and progress.

Getting involved as a nurse in clinical research

Nurses play an essential role in the medical field, not only in direct patient care, but also as a crucial link in the clinical research process. Their practical knowledge of patient care and proximity to patients make them ideally placed to influence and conduct research. Here is an exploration of the nurse's involvement in clinical research.

1. The role of the research nurse:
Nurses can play several roles in research, including as data collectors, coordinators of clinical studies or even principal investigators, designing and conducting studies.

2. Training and skills required:
Involvement in clinical research often requires additional training. Courses in research methodology, bioethics and statistics can be particularly useful. Some nurses go on to do a master's or doctorate to further their research skills.

3. Develop relevant research questions:
Thanks to their day-to-day clinical experience, nurses are well placed to identify gaps in knowledge or current practices. Formulating these questions can be the first step towards a clinical study.

4. Data collection:
Nurses are often on the front line when it comes to collecting data, whether through clinical observations, taking samples or interviewing patients. This proximity to the field is essential for obtaining reliable and relevant data.

5. Ethics and consent:
Nurses play a central role in obtaining informed consent from patients taking part in a study. They ensure that the patient understands the research, its risks and its potential benefits.

6. Interdisciplinary collaboration:
Involvement in research often means working closely with doctors, pharmacists, statisticians and other health professionals.

7. Dissemination of results:
Nurses involved in research can also take part in writing articles, presenting their work at conferences or taking part in training workshops for their peers.

8. Impact on clinical practice:
Ultimately, the aim of clinical research is to improve patient care. By translating the results of research into clinical practice, nurses play a decisive role in the continuous improvement of care.

Nurses' involvement in clinical research enriches the field of healthcare. Their unique perspective, combined with in-depth training, can lead to discoveries that directly influence the quality of care and well-being of patients. Every nurse, whether novice or experienced, has the potential to make a significant contribution to research and, ultimately, to the health and quality of life of the patients they serve.

Chapter 16:
CONTINUING EDUCATION
AND SPECIALISATION

Training courses post-basic for nurses

After graduating as a nurse, there are many post-basic training opportunities available to professionals wishing to specialise, deepen certain skills or develop their career. Here is an overview of post-basic training courses for nurses.

1. Specialised training:
There are several specialities available to nurses, enabling them to acquire expertise in a specific field.

Nurse anaesthetist (IADE): This training enables nurses to specialise in anaesthesia, intensive care and medical emergencies.

Operating theatre nurse (IBODE): Specialisation in the surgical field, focusing on assisting the surgeon and caring for the patient in the operating theatre.

Nursery nurse: Focused on caring for children, from newborns to adolescents.

Occupational health nurse: This speciality trains nurses in the prevention of occupational risks and the promotion of health in the workplace.

2. Master's degree in nursing:
It is an academic course that provides nurses with skills in research, project management and leadership in the healthcare field.

3. Management and leadership:
Training courses are available for those wishing to progress to positions such as nurse manager, director of care or team leader.

4. Short continuing training courses:
The aim of these courses is to enhance specific skills, such as pain management, palliative care, wound and scar treatment, gerontology, etc.

5. Training in psychotherapy:
For nurses wishing to specialise in mental health, training in psychotherapy, counselling or specific techniques (such as cognitive behavioural therapy) may be relevant.

6. University diplomas (DU) and inter-university diplomas (DIU):
Universities offer many DU and DIU courses in various fields such as oncology, diabetology, public health, medical ethics, etc.

7. Training abroad:
Nurses can also opt for post-basic training abroad to acquire new skills or a different approach to nursing.

The world of healthcare is constantly changing, and continuing education is a key element in staying up to date and providing the best possible care. Post-basic training courses offer nurses the opportunity to specialise, develop their careers and meet the changing needs of the population.

The value of certification
in geriatrics and dementia

Geriatrics, a science dedicated to the medical care of the elderly, and dementia, a multifaceted neurocognitive disorder, are areas of crucial importance in the current context of an ageing population. Certification in geriatrics and dementia is therefore of considerable value, both to the healthcare professional and to society as a whole. Here is an overview of this value.

1. Professional recognition:
Obtaining certification testifies to specific expertise. It can set a professional apart in a competitive environment and open the door to specialised job opportunities.

2. Skills update:
Dementia and geriatrics are constantly evolving fields. Certification guarantees that the professional is up to date with the latest practices, treatments and research.

3. Quality assurance:
For patients, their families and employers, certification is a guarantee that the nurse or doctor has specialised training and skills, ensuring better quality of care.

4. Responding to specific needs:
Older people and those with dementia have unique needs. Specialised training enables a holistic approach, taking into account medical, social and emotional aspects.

5. Improved patient outcomes:
Certified professionals are often more effective in preventing common complications in the elderly and can offer more appropriate intervention strategies for people with dementia.

6. Developing interprofessional collaboration:
Professionals certified in geriatrics and dementia are often seen as resources within their establishments. They can facilitate teamwork, provide training and contribute to the development of care policies.

7. Professional development:
Specialisation can bring great professional satisfaction. Faced with complex challenges, certified carers often find deep meaning in their work, helping a vulnerable population.

8. Positioning for leadership:
With certification, healthcare professionals can position themselves as leaders in their field, influencing decisions, policy and research.

In a society where the prevalence of age-related illnesses, particularly dementia, is on the rise, certification in geriatrics and dementia is more relevant than ever. It not only represents a step forward for the individual professional, but also strengthens the overall capacity of the healthcare system to respond to the needs of an ageing population with competence, compassion and efficiency.

Keeping up to date with the latest practices and recommendations

In the medical and healthcare field, the importance of keeping abreast of the latest research, practices and recommendations cannot be underestimated. Medicine is constantly evolving, with technological advances, scientific discoveries and new protocols. Here are some ways and reasons to keep up to date.

1. Why it's essential:
   Quality of care: Offering the best possible care means knowing and applying the latest and most effective methods.

   Patient safety: Keeping abreast of the latest recommendations can prevent medical errors and complications.

   Evolution of the profession: With the emergence of new diseases and conditions, as well as new treatments, the medical profession is constantly changing.

   Professional recognition: Professionals who are up to date in their field are more respected by their peers and generally have more professional opportunities.

2. How to stay up to date:
   Reading scientific journals: Peer-reviewed medical journals are reliable sources of the latest research and recommendations.

   Conferences and seminars: These gatherings offer conferences on the latest advances and provide an opportunity to network with experts in the field.

   Ongoing training: Many professional bodies and associations offer continuing training to help professionals strengthen and update their skills.

   Discussion groups and specialist forums: Online medical forums and discussion groups can be excellent platforms for exchanging information and experiences.

   Professional networks: Regular interaction with colleagues and experts can provide fresh perspectives and updates on current practice.

   Digital applications and platforms: Many medical applications provide regular updates on guidelines, medicines and protocols.

   Books and manuals: Although literature can quickly become obsolete in certain specialities, it remains a valuable resource for furthering knowledge.

3. Overcoming obstacles:

- **Lack of time**: It's crucial to set aside time on a regular basis to devote to professional updating, even if this means sacrificing other activities.
- **Information overload**: Given the volume of information available, it is essential to develop a strategy for filtering out what is most relevant and reliable.
- **Costs**: Attending conferences or buying subscriptions can be expensive, but think of it as an investment in your career. Many associations offer reduced rates or subsidies for continuing education.

Keeping up to date with the latest practices and recommendations is not just a professional obligation, but a duty to patients. In a constantly changing world, keeping up to date ensures that the level of care provided is the best possible, benefiting both the healthcare professional and those they serve.

Chapter 17:
PHARMACOLOGY AND ALZHEIMER'S DISEASE

Commonly prescribed medicines and their mode of action

Alzheimer's disease is a neurodegenerative disorder for which there is currently no cure. However, certain drugs have been developed to treat the cognitive and behavioural symptoms associated with the disease. Although these drugs cannot halt the progression of the disease, they can help improve patients' quality of life and slow the deterioration of certain cognitive functions.

1. Cholinesterase inhibitors:
    Donepezil (Aricept): Used to treat mild to moderate symptoms of Alzheimer's disease. It works by increasing levels of a neurotransmitter called acetylcholine, which is reduced in people with Alzheimer's disease.
    Rivastigmine (Exelon): Also used to treat mild to moderate symptoms. It works in the same way as Donepezil.
    Galantamine (Reminyl): This drug is prescribed for mild to moderate forms of the disease. It also works by increasing acetylcholine levels in the brain.
2. NMDA receptor antagonist:
    Memantine (Ebixa, Namenda): This is a treatment for moderate to severe symptoms of Alzheimer's disease. Instead of targeting acetylcholine, it works by regulating the activity of glutamate, another neurotransmitter. When produced in excess, glutamate can lead to brain cell death.

3. Medication to treat non-cognitive symptoms:

- **Antipsychotics**: These can be used to treat symptoms such as aggression, agitation or hallucinations. Examples include risperidone (Risperdal), olanzapine (Zyprexa) and quetiapine (Seroquel). However, these drugs can have significant side effects, particularly in the elderly.
- **Antidepressants**: These can be prescribed to treat the depressive symptoms often associated with Alzheimer's disease. Examples include sertraline (Zoloft) or citalopram (Celexa).
- **Anxiolytics**: Used to treat anxiety, drugs such as lorazepam (Ativan) and diazepam (Valium) may be prescribed, although they should be used with caution because of the risk of side effects.

It is crucial to note that the response to these drugs can vary from patient to patient. What's more, all these drugs can have side effects, some of which can be serious. This is why regular medical supervision is essential when taking these drugs. Decisions about medication should be taken in consultation with a doctor specialising in the treatment of dementia or Alzheimer's disease.

Managing side effects

Treating patients with Alzheimer's disease is not limited to managing cognitive symptoms. Often, the drugs prescribed can have side effects. For nurses, it is essential to be aware of these effects, to recognise them quickly, and to intervene accordingly, while educating the family and the patient themselves.

1. Identification of side effects:
First and foremost, it is essential to be aware of the common side effects associated with each drug. These can range from mild nausea to more serious reactions.

2. Regular monitoring:
Clinical observation: Monitor changes in behaviour, state of consciousness, mobility, nutrition, swallowing and other vital functions.
Questioning: Regularly ask patients how they are feeling, even if communication may be limited.

3. Proactive management:
Nausea and vomiting: These symptoms can be common, particularly with cholinesterase inhibitors. Taking the medicine with food may help. If the problem persists, it may be necessary to review the dosage or change the medication.
Diarrhoea or constipation: A balanced, high-fibre diet with adequate hydration can help prevent these symptoms. Mild laxatives may be considered if necessary.
Fatigue or weakness: Adjusting the time you take your medication, such as taking it in the evening, may be beneficial.

4. Management of neuropsychiatric side effects:
Some drugs, particularly antipsychotics, can cause symptoms such as agitation, insomnia or even hallucinations. In these cases, a reassessment of the need for the medication is essential. Sometimes, a dose adjustment or a change of medication may be necessary.

5. Family education:
Families need to be informed about potential side effects, how to recognise them and what to do if they are noticed. Open communication is essential.

6. Working with the medical team:
Work closely with the doctor, pharmacist and other members of the medical team. They can provide advice, adjust dosages or recommend alternatives.

7. Ethical considerations:
It is essential to always put the patient's interests first. If a drug causes more harm than good, its usefulness needs to be reassessed.

Managing side effects requires vigilance, patience and effective communication. The nurse, as the central pillar of patient care, plays a crucial role in ensuring that medicines improve quality of life without causing further harm.

New tracks
and experimental treatments

The medical world is constantly evolving, and Alzheimer's disease is no exception. Researchers around the world are working hard to discover new treatments, and some of these experimental developments offer a glimmer of hope for the future. For a healthcare professional, it is essential to stay informed and to be open to the integration of new methods or medicines into the care plan.

1. Gene therapies:
The idea is to use vectors to introduce or modulate the expression of specific genes that could play a role in the progression of the disease. Although still in its infancy, advances in gene therapy could open new doors in the fight against Alzheimer's.

2. Immunotherapy:
The aim of these treatments is to stimulate the immune system to target beta-amyloid proteins, considered to be at

the origin of the plaques characteristic of the disease. Monoclonal antibodies are at the forefront of this research.

3. Peptide-based treatment:
Some researchers are working on peptides designed to inhibit the formation of beta-amyloid plaques or to encourage their breakdown.

4. Electromagnetic stimulation:
The idea is to use electromagnetic fields to stimulate certain parts of the brain, in the hope of improving cognitive function and slowing the progression of the disease.

5. Multimodal approach:
Instead of targeting a single aspect of the disease, this method combines several interventions to address the different mechanisms involved in Alzheimer's disease.

6. Modulation of the microbiome:
Research has shown a connection between gut health and the brain, leading scientists to explore how altering the gut microbiome could influence Alzheimer's disease.

7. Stem cell therapies:
By using stem cells to replace damaged or dying neurons, it may be possible to restore some cognitive function.

8. Repurposed medicines:
Drugs initially developed for other conditions are being studied for their potential to treat Alzheimer's. For example, certain anti-diabetic drugs are being examined for their neuroprotective effects.

It is crucial to understand that many of these treatments are still at the experimental stage, and it will be some time before they become widely used, if they ever co. Nevertheless, they embody the innovation and determination of the scientific community to seek answers to one of the most pressing questions in modern medicine. For nurses, keeping abreast of these advances not only helps to improve care, but also brings hope and encouragement to patients and their families.

Chapter 18:
SPIRITUALITY AND CARE

The importance of spirituality in Alzheimer's patients

Spirituality is often an essential aspect of human life, influencing our understanding of ourselves, our place in the universe and our relationship with others. For people with Alzheimer's disease, spirituality can play a fundamental role in their overall well-being, quality of life and ability to cope with their condition.

1. Anchoring and identity:
Despite the cognitive losses and personality changes that can occur with Alzheimer's disease, spirituality often remains an intact part of an individual's identity. Rituals, prayers or familiar songs can remind a person of who they are and where they come from, providing a sense of continuity and connection to their past.

2. Comfort and peace:
Spirituality can offer immense comfort, particularly at times of confusion or distress. Spiritual rituals, prayer or meditation can bring a sense of peace, order and serenity in the face of the challenges of illness.

3. Strengthening community links:
Participation in spiritual or religious activities can help patients maintain social links, whether within a congregation, prayer group or other community groups. These connections can reduce feelings of isolation and strengthen a sense of belonging.

4. Emotional expression:
Spirituality often offers a space where emotions, even those that are difficult to express, can be recognised and validated. Feelings such as grief, frustration, anger or hope can be channelled through prayer, meditation or other spiritual practices.

5. Perspective on the disease:
Certain spiritual or religious traditions can offer a perspective on suffering, illness or decline, helping individuals and their families to find meaning or purpose in their experience.

6. Support for carers:
Spirituality supports not only the patient, but also their family and carers. It can offer resources for managing stress, sadness and burnout, and can be a crucial part of the bereavement process.

7. Preparing for the end of life:
Spirituality can help to address issues related to death, the afterlife and other existential concerns. It can guide individuals and their families through the end-of-life stages, providing a framework for understanding and accepting death.

For nurses working with Alzheimer's patients, recognising and respecting each individual's spirituality is essential. This means listening actively, asking questions about spiritual needs and preferences, and incorporating these into the care plan. Giving space to spirituality can enrich the patient's experience and support a deeper quality of life, even in the midst of the challenges of Alzheimer's disease.

Integrating spiritual care in practice

Integrating the spiritual dimension into nursing care, particularly for Alzheimer's patients, means embracing the totality of human experience. Spirituality, whether linked to a religious tradition or taking a more universal form, goes to the heart of what it means to be human. For many, it is the source of strength, comfort and meaning, particularly in the face of challenges such as illness.

1. Spiritual evaluation:
One of the first steps in integrating spiritual care is to conduct a spiritual assessment. This may involve asking questions about the patient's beliefs, practices, rituals and spiritual needs. Such an assessment allows care to be tailored to the patient's spiritual needs.

2. Creating a sacred space:
Even in a medical environment, creating a small space dedicated to prayer, meditation or other spiritual practices can be beneficial. It can be as simple as a corner of the room with a few spiritual objects, such as a sacred image, a rosary or a candle.

3. Encouraging spiritual practice:
If the patient has a regular practice, such as prayer or meditation, it is important to support and enable them to access it. This may involve setting up a prayer schedule or facilitating access to resources such as sacred texts.

4. Working with chaplains or spiritual guides:
A partnership with the hospital chaplaincy service or with external spiritual guides can help meet the complex spiritual needs of patients. These professionals can offer support, rituals and ceremonies tailored to the patient's situation.

5. Active and empathetic listening:
Listening is one of the most powerful tools in spiritual care. Patients often need to talk about their fears, hopes and beliefs. Empathetic, non-judgemental listening can offer great comfort.

6. Continuing education:
It is essential for nurses to learn about different spiritual and religious traditions on a regular basis, so that they can approach patients with respect and understanding.

7. Self-care and introspection:
Nurses themselves can benefit from integrating spirituality into their own lives. Connecting with one's own spirituality can help to manage stress, avoid burnout and provide more empathetic care.

Addressing spiritual needs is an essential facet of holistic care. For Alzheimer's patients, whose identity and memory may be in decline, rituals and spiritual beliefs can provide an anchor, a sense of continuity and connection. As nurses, our role is to recognise, honour and support this dimension of the human experience, enriching our practice and the lives of our patients.

Respect for beliefs and customs

Patients with Alzheimer's disease, although faced with cognitive challenges, retain a profound identity rooted in their life experiences, values and beliefs. Nurses have a responsibility not only to provide medical care, but also to recognise and respect the beliefs and customs that form the fabric of a patient's life. Here's how such sensitivity enriches clinical care.

1. Importance of beliefs and customs:
Spirituality and cultural customs provide meaning, structure and continuity for many people. These elements often play a key role in their understanding of health, illness and healing. Acknowledging their importance is essential for comprehensive and respectful care.

2. Initial assessment of beliefs and customs:
As soon as patients are admitted, it is crucial to gather information about their religious or cultural beliefs and practices. This ensures that care is aligned with these essential aspects of their identity.

3. Inclusion in the care plan:
Once beliefs and customs have been identified, they need to be incorporated into the care plan. This may involve setting up a special diet, taking into account holy days or providing a space for prayer.

4. Working with families:
Families play a central role in maintaining and passing on beliefs and customs. By establishing an open dialogue with them, nurses can better understand and respond to the patient's specific needs.

5. Flexibility and adaptation:
It is essential to approach care with a flexible attitude, ready to adapt to the patient's cultural and spiritual needs. This could mean shifting medication times during Ramadan or allowing traditional healing rituals in conjunction with medical treatment.

6. Education and training:
It is crucial that nurses receive ongoing training in respecting different beliefs and customs. Understanding and respecting cultural and religious diversity builds trust and improves the quality of care.

7. Personal reflection:
Nurses also need to be aware of their own beliefs and prejudices. Regular introspection and a commitment to professional development can help to provide non-judgemental care.

Respect for beliefs and customs is not just an add-on to nursing care, it is a fundamental dimension. Patients, in all their diversity, deserve care that recognises and honours their individuality. By focusing on respect and understanding, nurses can strengthen the bond of trust with their patients and families, providing truly holistic, person-centred care.

Chapter 19:
CULTURAL DIVERSITY
IN AN ALZHEIMER'S UNIT

Understanding cultural influence
on the perception of illness

Culture profoundly shapes the way we perceive the world around us, including our understanding and experience of health and illness. For a nurse working in an Alzheimer's unit, understanding these cultural nuances is essential to providing individualised and empathetic care.

1. Cultural beliefs and Alzheimer's disease:
Each culture has its own beliefs about the origin and cause of illness. In some cultures, dementia may be seen as a natural consequence of ageing, while in others it may be interpreted as a curse or the result of past actions. These beliefs have a profound influence on how individuals and their families perceive and react to a diagnosis.

2. The role of carers in different cultures:
In some traditions, the family is expected to take on a large part of the care responsibilities. This expectation may be in contrast to other cultures where the use of outside care is the norm. Understanding these dynamics helps the nurse to navigate interactions with families and support their decisions.

3. Communication and stigmatisation:
Alzheimer's disease and other forms of dementia can be stigmatised in some cultures, leading families to avoid talking about it or to hide the diagnosis. This stigma can

influence how quickly care is sought and how well the patient is integrated into the community.

4. Rituals, routines and customs:
Daily rituals, prayer routines and other cultural customs can have a profound influence on patients' well-being. Respecting and integrating these practices into the care plan can help to soothe and guide patients, while preserving a sense of identity.

5. Alternative and complementary approaches:
Some cultures may favour traditional remedies or holistic approaches to managing the symptoms of illness. Although these methods do not replace medical treatment, they can offer comfort and familiarity to patients.

6. Importance of cultural training:
Carers need to be trained in cultural competence, an approach that values diversity, encourages personal reflection and promotes continuous learning about different cultural perspectives.

Culture, in all its richness and complexity, plays a central role in how we understand and approach Alzheimer's disease. By approaching each patient and their family with an open mind, asking questions and seeking to understand, nurses can transcend cultural barriers and provide truly personalised and caring care.

Adapting care
according to cultural background

Dealing with Alzheimer's disease involves not only medical expertise, but also the sensitivity with which a healthcare professional approaches and interacts with the patient. This becomes even more relevant when we take into account the rich fabric of cultural diversity that makes up our society. Adapting care to the cultural background is an approach that recognises and respects this diversity, ensuring that every patient is treated with dignity and understanding.

1. Listening for understanding:
Rather than applying a one-size-fits-all approach, it is crucial to actively listen to patients and their families to understand their values, beliefs and expectations. This active listening serves as a guide to personalising the care plan.

2. Recognition of customs and rituals:
Whether it's a daily ritual, a prayer routine, or traditional meals, these customs can have a profound meaning for the patient. Incorporating these rituals into daily care can provide a sense of normality and comfort.

3. Working with the family:
The family often plays a central role in patient care, particularly in cultures where caring for the elderly is highly valued. Working closely with the family, while respecting their wishes and preferences, can enhance the quality of care.

4. Respect for traditional medical beliefs:
Some cultures may favour traditional remedies or alternative approaches. Although these methods need to be evaluated in terms of safety and efficacy, showing respect and openness to these practices builds trust between carer and patient.

5. Language barriers:
Language can be a major barrier to care. Using interpreters or technological tools to facilitate communication can considerably improve the quality of care and avoid misunderstandings.

6. Cultural competence training:
It is imperative that nurses receive ongoing training in cultural competence, helping them to understand the specific nuances of each culture and to adapt their care accordingly.

7. Sensitivity to cultural taboos:
Some cultures may have specific taboos relating to physical contact, modesty or other aspects of care. Being aware of and respectful of these sensitivities can avoid offending the patient or their family.

Adapting care to cultural backgrounds is not simply a question of politeness or convenience. It is an approach deeply rooted in respect for human dignity, recognising that each individual is the bearer of a history, a culture and an identity that deserve to be honoured. By emphasising individuality and personalisation, carers can offer truly holistic care, where the patient is always at the heart of the care process.

Communicating effectively across language barriers

In today's medical landscape, healthcare professionals frequently face communication challenges that are exacerbated by language barriers. Alzheimer's disease, with its grip on memory and cognition, amplifies these challenges even further. For nurses working in Alzheimer's units, skilfully navigating these language barriers is essential to ensuring effective, empathetic care.

1. The importance of non-verbal communication:
When words fail or cannot be understood, body language takes over. A reassuring smile, a gentle touch or a simple gesture of listening can convey a message of

understanding and support. These non-verbal nuances can often act as a bridge between nurse and patient when language is a barrier.

2. Use of professional interpreters:
Interpreting services, whether in person, by telephone or via apps, can be invaluable. A professional interpreter is not just a translator of words, but also a translator of cultural context, ensuring that nuances and subtleties are preserved.

3. Technological tools:
Today there is a wide range of applications and tools that can facilitate translation in real time. Although these tools do not completely replace a human interpreter, they can be a great help during rapid interactions or when there are no interpreters available.

4. Pictograms and images:
Images or pictograms can be used to illustrate actions, needs or feelings. These visual tools can bridge the language gap, particularly in situations where it is crucial to understand the patient's immediate needs.

5. Training and awareness-raising:
For nurses, training in intercultural communication techniques and strategies for overcoming language barriers is vital. This training prepares them to be more competent and confident in their interactions with patients from different linguistic backgrounds.

6. Encouraging language learning:
Fostering an environment where nurses are encouraged to learn key phrases in several languages can strengthen communication. Even a simple greeting or word of thanks in the patient's mother tongue can create a sense of belonging and respect.

7. Appropriate documentation:
Written information, whether in the form of medical instructions, information sheets or guidelines, should be available in several languages to meet the needs of a diverse range of patients.

Language barriers, while challenging, need not be insurmountable obstacles in medical care. With the right resources, the right training and a dose of creativity and empathy, nurses can ensure effective communication, boosting patients' confidence and well-being. Ultimately, the desire to connect and understand transcends words and is based on the shared humanity between carer and patient.

Chapter 20:
ALTERNATIVE AND COMPLEMENTARY THERAPIES

Aromatherapy, acupressure and other non-traditional methods

Throughout the ages, mankind has constantly sought ways to heal, soothe and comfort. Beyond the boundaries of conventional medicine, many alternative therapies have emerged and been integrated into clinical practice to offer a holistic approach to care. In the context of Alzheimer's disease, aromatherapy, acupressure and other non-traditional techniques are emerging as promising avenues for improving patients' quality of life.

1. Aromatherapy: the influence of fragrance on the mind
Aromatherapy uses essential oils extracted from plants to stimulate well-being. In Alzheimer's patients, certain oils, such as lavender or rosemary, have been shown to have calming or memory-stimulating effects. When diffused or massaged, these oils can help reduce anxiety, improve sleep and even stimulate certain memories.

2. Acupressure: well-placed pressure
Derived from acupuncture, acupressure is a technique that uses finger pressure on specific points on the body to balance energies. It can help reduce restlessness, improve sleep and reduce pain. The main advantage is that it does not require the use of needles, which makes it more acceptable to some patients.

3. Reflexology

Reflexology, which often focuses on the feet, postulates that different points correspond to other parts or functions of our body. Gentle, targeted pressure on these points can offer relaxation and relief from certain ailments, helping to calm agitated Alzheimer's patients.

4. Sound therapy

Whether using Tibetan bowls, tuning forks or other instruments, sound therapy aims to harmonise body and mind. For Alzheimer's patients, these sounds can trigger memories, reduce anxiety or simply offer a moment of escape.

5. Chromotherapy

This therapy uses colours to influence mood and emotions. Certain colours, such as blue or green, can have a calming effect, while others, such as yellow or red, can stimulate and energise.

While these techniques do not claim to cure Alzheimer's disease, they can offer moments of respite, relaxation and improved quality of life. It is essential for carers to be trained in these practices, to understand them and to integrate them judiciously into the care pathway, always respecting the patient's preferences and safety. Combined with conventional treatments, these non-traditional methods pave the way for holistic, rich and diversified care.

Evaluation of effectiveness and limitations

Every Alzheimer's patient is unique, with symptoms, history and response to treatment varying greatly. While non-traditional techniques such as aromatherapy or acupressure show benefits in some cases, it is imperative to evaluate them rigorously to better understand their potential and limitations.

1. Systematic assessment

The importance of documentation cannot be underestimated. Before introducing an alternative therapy, it is crucial to establish a baseline of the patient's symptoms, behaviours and general well-being. Then, any changes, positive or negative, must be recorded regularly and conscientiously to provide a clear overview of the effectiveness of the technique.

2. Clinical trials and studies

Evaluation must not be limited to anecdotal observation. The introduction of unconventional techniques into clinical practice must be based on solid studies, clinical trials or meta-analyses that attest to their effectiveness.

3. The benefits observed

Many patients and their families report a marked improvement in quality of life with some of these techniques. Whether it's a reduction in anxiety, an improvement in sleep or an increase in lucid moments, these precious moments can contribute greatly to general well-being.

4. Limits and precautions

It is equally important to recognise that not all of these methods will work for every patient. In addition, some may interfere with drug treatments or be contraindicated due to specific conditions. For example, some essential oils may be too strong for patients with sensitive skin, and acupressure may not be recommended for those with circulatory problems.

5. The importance of proper training

One of the major risks of incorporating non-traditional techniques is incorrect implementation. Carers need to be properly trained and understand both theory and practice in order to deliver these therapies safely.

As traditional medicine continues to evolve in its understanding and management of Alzheimer's disease, the opening up to complementary modalities offers a wider range of tools to improve patients' quality of life. However, as with any intervention, rigorous evaluation of their effectiveness and limitations is essential to ensure safe, respectful and genuinely beneficial care.

Integration into the care plan

The management of Alzheimer's disease requires a holistic approach, encompassing both traditional medical interventions and, where appropriate, complementary modalities. Integrating these different strategies into a structured care plan is crucial to ensuring a coherent, individualised and patient-centred approach.
1. Initial assessment of the patient
Before drawing up a care plan, it is essential to carry out a full assessment of the patient. This assessment should cover not only the stage of the disease and the symptoms, but also the patient's preferences, medical history, cultural and spiritual background, and the needs and wishes of the family.

2. Setting care plan objectives
The objectives must be clear, measurable and tailored to each patient. For example, if a patient has significant anxiety, one objective could be to reduce these episodes through aromatherapy or relaxation sessions.

3. Selection of appropriate interventions
Once the objectives have been set, the next step is to determine which interventions will be most beneficial. If a

patient has shown an interest in music in the past, music therapy could be integrated as a means of cognitive stimulation.

4. Coordination with the care team

All members of the care team, from doctors to care assistants, must be informed of the care plan and understand their role in implementing it. This coordination ensures that the patient receives consistent care, regardless of who is involved.

5. Ongoing assessment and adjustments

A care plan is never static. It must be regularly reviewed and adjusted according to the progress of the disease, responses to interventions and any changes in the patient's preferences or needs.

6. Family involvement

The family plays a crucial role in the management of Alzheimer's disease. Their involvement can vary, ranging from simple information to active participation in certain interventions, such as art therapy sessions or daily walks.

Integrating different treatment modalities into a care plan for a patient with Alzheimer's disease can seem complex. However, with careful assessment, detailed planning and effective communication within the care team, it is possible to create an environment rich in interventions that are tailored to and beneficial for the patient. It is only with this integrated approach that the complex needs of these patients and their families can truly be met.

Chapter 21:
SEXUALITY IN ALZHEIMER PATIENTS

The needs and challenges of sexuality

Sexuality, although often neglected in discussions about the care of patients with Alzheimer's disease, remains an essential component of human identity and well-being. The needs and challenges associated with sexuality in the context of Alzheimer's disease are complex and require a sensitive, respectful and understanding approach.

1. Recognising the validity of sexual needs
Even as the disease progresses, many patients retain sexual needs and desires. It is essential for healthcare staff to recognise that these feelings are natural and valid, while ensuring that the patient is able to give informed consent.

2. Communication difficulties
One of the major challenges is the gradual decline in the patient's ability to communicate their wishes, limitations and needs. This requires particular care on the part of carers to interpret non-verbal behaviours and ensure the patient's well-being.

3. Inappropriate sexual behaviour
Some patients may develop inappropriate sexual behaviour as a result of impaired judgement and inhibitions. In such cases, it is crucial to approach the situation with compassion, trying to understand the underlying cause of the behaviour and putting in place strategies to manage it.

4. The role of family and friends
Patients' spouses and partners may experience conflicting feelings, oscillating between the desire to maintain intimacy

with their loved one and grief at the gradual loss of the person they knew. Psychological support is essential to help them navigate this delicate area.

5. Questions of consent
The cognitive decline associated with Alzheimer's disease raises significant concerns about consent in the context of sexual relationships. Staff training and clear guidelines on assessing capacity to consent are essential.

6. Therapeutic approaches
For some patients, specific therapies, such as couple therapy or sex therapy, may be beneficial. These interventions can help treat sexual problems arising in the context of the disease.

Sexuality in the context of Alzheimer's disease presents many challenges, but it is intrinsically linked to the patient's dignity, identity and well-being. Appropriate, respectful and well-informed care can enable patients and their partners to experience their sexuality in a safe and fulfilling way.

Manage inappropriate sexual behaviour

The onset of inappropriate sexual behaviour in Alzheimer's patients can be a major source of concern for carers, families and other patients. This issue, although delicate, is an aspect of care that carers need to address with sensitivity, professionalism and empathy.

1. Understanding the origins of behaviour
Inappropriate sexual behaviour can be the result of a variety of factors, including :

    Loss of inhibitions due to deterioration of the frontal lobes.

   Misinterpretation of social signals or confusion between people.

   Unmet needs, such as the need for physical contact or affection.

2. Prevention and a safe environment

   Make sure that communal areas are supervised and that patients have a private space for their personal needs.

   Encourage structured activities that reduce boredom and frustration, which can lead to inappropriate behaviour.

   Provide specific training for staff to anticipate and manage these behaviours.

3. Non-confrontational interventions

When inappropriate behaviour occurs :

   Divert the patient's attention to another activity.

   Respond calmly and gently, and avoid expressing anger or frustration.

   Explain the appropriate limits simply and clearly.

4. Communication with families

It is essential to involve the family in the management process. Inform them of the occurrence of such behaviour and reassure them of the measures taken to deal with it. This transparency builds trust between the healthcare team and the patient's family.

5. Medical reassessment

   Consult your GP to determine whether there are any underlying medical causes, such as a urinary tract infection, that may be contributing to this behaviour.

   Review current medications to ensure they are not exacerbating the problem.

6. Staff support and training
Staff must be trained to recognise and respond to inappropriate sexual behaviour. Debriefing sessions and support groups can help staff deal with the stress and emotions associated with these situations.

Although challenging, inappropriate sexual behaviour can be successfully managed through a combination of preventive approaches, tailored interventions and open communication. Respect for the dignity of the patient, while ensuring the safety of all, must always be at the heart of our concerns.

Education and awareness the care team

In the complex and demanding environment of an Alzheimer's unit, ongoing education and awareness-raising for the care team are essential. More than simply passing on technical skills, this involves developing a deeper understanding of the specific challenges of the disease, strengthening empathy and refining intervention techniques.

1. Understanding Alzheimer's disease
    Biological basis: Understanding the underlying neurological mechanisms, the areas of the brain affected and the associated symptoms.
    Psychosocial impact: Recognising how the disease affects the patient's relationships, self-esteem and well-being.
2. Person-centred approach techniques
    Emphasis on the patient's dignity, preferences and individual needs.
    Remember that, behind the illness, there is a person with a history, likes and dislikes and an identity of their own.

3. Effective communication with patients
   - Learn to use simple, clear, repetitive language.
   - Know the techniques for engaging, reassuring and defusing tense situations.
4. Identifying and managing difficult behaviour
   - Understanding common triggers and warning signs.
   - Non-pharmacological intervention techniques to manage agitation, aggression and depression, among others.
5. Interdisciplinary collaboration
   - Valuing the role of each member of the team, from doctors to care assistants.
   - Interprofessional communication techniques for coherent, coordinated care.
6. Importance of the emotional health of the team
   - Recognising the signs of burnout and prevention methods.
   - Promoting goodwill and mutual support.
7. Further training
   - Keep abreast of advances in research, treatments and best practice.
   - Encourage participation in workshops, conferences and specialist training courses.
8. Interaction with families
   - Techniques for communicating effectively with relatives, managing their expectations and involving them in care.

Education and awareness are not mere formalities: they are the foundation of high-quality, respectful and effective care. By investing in continuing education and awareness-raising, facilities can ensure that every patient receives appropriate care, while the care team is supported and valued in its essential role.

Chapter 22:
THERAPEUTIC AND RECREATIONAL ACTIVITIES

The importance of social commitment and stimulation

Social involvement and stimulation are two essential elements in the care of patients suffering from Alzheimer's disease. While this disease can often seem to isolate people from their environment, these two approaches aim to break this solitude and maintain the patient's quality of life as much as possible. Let's take a closer look at their importance and benefits.

The social nature of human beings
Man is, by nature, a social being. Our experiences, memories and relationships are the cornerstones of our identity. For Alzheimer's patients, these connections may fade, but the fundamental need for connection remains. Social engagement offers an opportunity to rekindle these bonds, stimulate memories and strengthen the sense of belonging.

The benefits of cognitive stimulation
Stimulation, whether cognitive, sensory or physical, is like gymnastics for the brain.
It has the effect of :

> **Slowing the progression of symptoms**: Although there is no cure for the disease, regular stimulation can help preserve certain cognitive functions for longer.

- **Boosting self-esteem**: Taking part in stimulating activities and successfully completing certain tasks, however simple, can provide a sense of achievement.

Social activities as a vehicle for well-being
Activities such as discussion groups, singing, board games or group outings can have many benefits:
- **Reduced sense of isolation**: Feeling part of a community or group can reduce feelings of loneliness and isolation.
- **Emotional stimulation**: The positive emotions generated by social interaction can have a positive impact on general well-being.

The inestimable value of routine
Familiar routines, combined with regular stimulation, can provide a sense of normality and predictability for patients, who can often feel disorientated and anxious.

Social engagement and stimulation are not mere distractions; they are essential to the quality of life of Alzheimer's patients. In a world that can sometimes seem blurred and disorientating, these moments of connection and activation can offer a sense of purpose, joy and belonging. They remind these patients, and those around them, that behind the disease there is still a person with needs, desires and a capacity to feel and engage.

Examples of adapted activities
at different stages of the disease

Adapting activities as Alzheimer's disease progresses is crucial to ensuring patients' well-being, comfort and involvement. The choice of activities should take into account the stage of the disease, individual preferences and the patient's remaining abilities. Let's look at some examples of activities for each stage.

1. Early stage:
At this stage, people with Alzheimer's disease are often still independent in many activities of daily living. The activities are aimed primarily at stimulating their minds and maintaining their existing skills.

- **Reading**: Encourage reading newspapers, magazines and novels.
- **Board games**: chess, scrabble, card games.
- **Craft activities**: painting, knitting, gardening.
- **Listening to music and dancing**: Choose songs they like.
- **Intellectual activities**: crosswords, sudoku, puzzles.

2. Moderate stage:
At this stage, the disease progresses, and more marked cognitive deficits appear. Activities are simplified, but still offer a sense of fulfilment.

- **Simple cooking**: bake cookies, decorate cakes.
- **Looking at photos**: leafing through photo albums, reminiscing.
- **Singing**: Sing traditional songs or nursery rhymes.
- **Adapted physical exercise**: walking, tai chi, gentle yoga.
- **Sensory activities**: light gardening, handling textured objects.

3. Advanced stage:
At this stage, verbal communication is often limited, and sensory needs become paramount. Activities are aimed primarily at providing comfort, calming and creating a sense of security.

- **Touch therapy**: Gentle massages with scented lotions.

- **Music therapy**: Listening to soothing or familiar melodies.
- **Art therapy**: finger painting, modelling with modelling clay.
- **Water therapy**: Relaxing hot baths or simple water games.
- **Light stimulation**: Look at soft lights or star projectors.

Each person with Alzheimer's disease is unique, and their preferences and abilities will vary. It is important to observe and listen carefully to the patient's reactions, adjust activities accordingly and always approach each activity with patience, empathy and respect. The key is to find ways of maintaining a connection, stimulating the brain and body, and offering moments of joy, peace and comfort at every stage of this disease.

Integration of volunteers and families

In addition to healthcare professionals, the commitment of families and volunteers plays a decisive role in supporting people with Alzheimer's disease. Their involvement can not only improve the patient's quality of life, but also lighten the workload of healthcare professionals. However, this integration requires a well-coordinated approach, based on training, communication and mutual respect.

1. The role of volunteers:
   - **Complementary services**: Volunteers can offer services that complement those of professionals, such as recreational activities, reading or simply companionship.
   - **Training**: For volunteers to be effective, it is crucial that they are trained in the specificities of Alzheimer's

disease, communication techniques and the limits of their role.

Coordination: Volunteers are expected to work closely with the care team, sharing observations and concerns and receiving advice and support.

2. Family commitment:

Personalised care: Families bring an intimate knowledge of the person, their preferences and their history. They can help personalise care and activities, making the experience more meaningful for the patient.

Emotional support: The presence of loved ones can reassure and soothe patients, reinforcing their sense of security and belonging.

Communication: Regular exchanges between the medical team and families are essential for sharing information, aligning expectations and collaborating on decision-making.

3. Establish protocols:

Orientation: Both volunteers and families should be given guidance on how the unit works, the rules to follow and how to interact appropriately with patients and staff.

Feedback: It is beneficial to hold regular meetings to gather feedback, share progress and discuss challenges.

Limits: While we value the commitment of volunteers and families, it is crucial to clearly define their limits to avoid any confusion or encroachment on professional roles.

Involving volunteers and families in the care of Alzheimer's patients is a team effort that requires coordination, respect and communication. When well managed, this collaboration can add immense value, enriching the lives of patients and supporting the incredible work of healthcare professionals.

Chapter 23:
ECONOMIC ISSUES ALZHEIMER CARE

The cost of care: a global perspective

Because of its complexity, duration and impact, Alzheimer's disease represents a financial challenge not only for patients' families, but also for the public and private healthcare systems. Understanding the overall cost of care is essential for anticipating, planning and allocating resources effectively.

1. Direct costs:
   - **Medical services: These** are costs incurred for medical consultations, hospitalisation, drug treatments, specialist therapies and other health services.
   - **Care at home and in institutions**: Hiring home carers or providing care in a specialist retirement home can represent a significant cost.
   - **Medical equipment**: From monitoring equipment to adapted bedding, these costs can add up quickly.
2. Indirect costs:
   - **Loss of income**: Families may have to reduce their working hours or even quit their jobs to care for a loved one with Alzheimer's disease.
   - **Social costs**: Stress, depression and exhaustion among carers can lead to additional costs in terms of mental health and well-being for families.
3. Cost to society:
   - **Healthcare systems**: Frequent hospital admissions, specialist consultations and long-term treatments are putting pressure on public finances.

Economic productivity: Reducing the working hours of carers, as well as the potential early withdrawal of patients from the labour market, can have an economic impact.

4. Mitigation strategies:

Insurance and cover: Specialised insurance policies can help cover certain costs, but it is essential to understand the terms and limits.

Early financial planning: Consulting a financial planner at the first signs of the disease can help establish a strategy for managing future costs.

Government support: Find out about the support and allowances available for Alzheimer's patients and their families.

Community initiatives: Some community programmes or NGOs offer low-cost or free services, such as support groups, workshops and adapted activities.

There is no denying that the cost of Alzheimer's care is substantial, but with a thorough understanding, early planning and access to appropriate resources, families can navigate this financial landscape with greater confidence and peace of mind.

Financing and medical cover

Care for Alzheimer's disease goes far beyond simple medical treatment. It involves a comprehensive approach, taking into account the clinical aspect, the patient's well-being, family support and, inevitably, the financial aspects. Understanding the different funding mechanisms and medical cover options is vital to ensure optimum care for the patient while preserving family resources.

1. The health insurance landscape:
   - **Public insurance**: In many countries, public health systems offer some cover for Alzheimer's patients. It is essential to find out about the eligibility criteria, the benefits covered and any reimbursement ceilings.
   - **Private insurance**: Depending on the policy, certain types of insurance may cover a significant proportion of the costs. However, clauses and exclusions vary. It is crucial to understand your insurance policy and to consider additional insurance policies specifically for long-term care or degenerative diseases.
2. Government aid and subsidies:
   - **National programmes**: Some countries have dedicated programmes to help Alzheimer's patients and their families financially, whether in the form of direct aid, tax exemptions or other support measures.
   - **Local initiatives**: Grants or funding may also be available at local level, through town councils or regional bodies.
3. Hidden costs:
   - **Non-reimbursed medicines**: Not all medicines are covered by insurance. It is vital to find out in advance and consider alternatives or medical assistance programmes.
   - **Non-conventional care**: Therapies such as music or art therapy can be beneficial, but are not always reimbursed. It is worth exploring community initiatives or NGOs that may offer these services at reduced cost or free of charge.
4. Long-term planning:
   - **Endowment funds**: Setting up an endowment fund or dedicated savings can help cover future costs and ensure continuity of care.
   - **Financial advice**: Consulting a financial expert, particularly one specialising in medical or long-term care, can help you navigate the complex financial landscape of Alzheimer's care.

5. Research and advocacy:

Keep up to date: Government policies, assistance programmes and insurance options are evolving. It's essential to keep abreast of the latest developments to maximise the cover and funding available.

Community involvement: Getting involved in associations or advocacy groups can not only provide support, but also positively influence policies and funding programmes.

The financing and medical coverage of Alzheimer's care requires a holistic vision, encompassing not only the immediate needs of the patient, but also the long-term implications for families. A proactive, informed and planned approach can facilitate this, ensuring the best possible quality of life for the patient while preserving the financial health of the family.

Economic value the specialist nurse

With their in-depth training and advanced skills, specialist nurses are an essential part of the medical landscape. In addition to their clinical role, specialist nurses have an economic value that is often underestimated, both for healthcare establishments and for the healthcare system as a whole. Let's look at the many facets of this economic value.

1. Reducing hospital costs:

Fewer readmissions: Thanks to specialised care and a patient-centred approach, the specialist nurse can help to reduce the number of readmissions, representing significant savings for hospitals.

Optimisation of resources: Thanks to their expertise, they are often able to manage complex cases efficiently, minimising hospital stays and the use of costly resources.

2. Improving the effectiveness of care:

Informed decision-making: The specialist nurse is often involved in ethics committees, think tanks or boards of directors, contributing to more strategic and economically beneficial decisions.

Training and mentoring: By training other nursing staff, they help to improve the overall skills of the team, resulting in more effective care and a reduction in costly medical errors.

3. Enhancing the value of outpatient care:

Home care: As healthcare needs evolve, more and more services are offered outside the hospital setting. The specialist nurse plays a central role in providing high-quality home care, thereby reducing the costs associated with lengthy hospital stays.

4. Research and innovation:

Participation in clinical research: Specialist nurses are often at the forefront of clinical studies, contributing to the development of best practice, which can lead to long-term savings.

Introduction of innovative technologies: Thanks to their advanced training, they are often the first to adopt and train other professionals in new technologies or techniques, optimising care and reducing costs.

5. Patient satisfaction:

Quality of care: Care provided by specialist nurses is often synonymous with superior quality, which increases patient satisfaction and can have positive economic implications, particularly in terms of patient retention and positive word-of-mouth.

6. Liaison with other health professionals:

Care coordination: The specialist nurse often acts as a bridge between different specialists, ensuring that the patient receives coordinated care, which can reduce duplication, unnecessary tests and other unnecessary costs.

The economic value of the specialist nurse extends far beyond their mere presence in the hospital or clinic. It is a combination of clinical expertise, innovation, training and coordination that collectively adds immense value to the entire healthcare system.

Chapter 24:
SUPPORT NETWORKS
AND AVAILABLE RESOURCES

Associations and organisations dedicated to Alzheimer's

In the vast world of healthcare, community support plays an essential role, providing patients, families and healthcare professionals with resources, training and advocacy. Among the many diseases affecting the world's population, Alzheimer's disease, with its complexity and multiple challenges, has prompted the creation of a large number of associations and organisations. These dedicated bodies play a major role in raising awareness, conducting research, supporting patients and families, and training healthcare professionals.

1. Raising awareness and advocacy:
   Global campaigns: Many organisations, such as the World Alzheimer's Association, are running global awareness campaigns, highlighting the importance of recognition and investment in Alzheimer's research.
   World Alzheimer's Day: Celebrated every year on 21 September, this day is dedicated to raising public awareness of Alzheimer's disease and its impact.
2. Research and development:
   Research funding: Organisations such as Alzheimer's Research UK and the Alzheimer's Association in the United States are actively funding promising research aimed at discovering more effective treatments and, ultimately, a cure.
   Conferences and symposia: These associations regularly organise conferences that bring together

researchers from all over the world, encouraging the sharing of knowledge and innovations.

3. Support for patients and families:

Helplines: Many organisations offer telephone helplines, enabling patients and families to obtain advice, support and information.

Support groups: These groups, often led by trained professionals or volunteers, offer a safe space to share, learn and find comfort.

4. Training and resources for professionals:

Workshops and seminars: These sessions are designed to help healthcare professionals keep abreast of the latest practices and discoveries in the management of Alzheimer's disease.

Publications and guidelines: Organisations often publish guides, brochures and other printed resources to educate and inform professionals about various aspects of the disease.

5. International collaboration:

Networks and partnerships: Organisations often work in networks, sharing resources, information and best practice across borders.

Exchange programmes: Some of these enable researchers and healthcare professionals to collaborate with their international counterparts, enriching their understanding and approach to the disease.

Alzheimer's associations and organisations play a fundamental role in the fight against the disease. Not only do they offer vital support to patients and their families, but they also make a significant contribution to research, education and global awareness. For healthcare professionals, they are invaluable allies, providing tools, resources and an essential support network.

Professional networks for nurses

The art of medicine, with its constant challenges, perpetual evolution and ethical imperatives, requires constant and effective collaboration between professionals. For nurses, joining and actively participating in professional networks is essential to keep up to date, share experiences, obtain support and contribute to the progress of the profession. Let's explore these networks and the importance of their role for the modern nurse.

1. The importance of professional networks:

    Updating and continuing education: The medical world is changing fast. The networks give nurses access to training, conferences and workshops to keep abreast of the latest practices.

    Sharing experiences: Clinical challenges often manifest themselves in a variety of ways. Exchanging with peers can provide advice, tips and new perspectives to improve care.

    Emotional and professional support: Nursing is a demanding profession. Networks offer a place to share concerns, find support and, sometimes, simply decompress.

2. Types of networks:

    Professional associations: Organisations such as the College of Nurses and the American Nurses Association offer their members professional development opportunities and resources, and defend nurses' rights.

    Specialist groups: For nurses working in specific fields, such as paediatrics, oncology or geriatrics, there are specialist groups focusing on these areas.

    Online platforms: Forums, social networking groups and dedicated sites allow nurses to connect virtually, sharing resources, stories and advice.

Local groups and workshops: Sometimes groups are formed at local level, organising meetings, exchange sessions and workshops to strengthen local skills and networks.

3. Getting actively involved:

    Attending events: Conferences, workshops and seminars offer opportunities not only for learning, but also for networking.

    Active contribution: Sharing articles, taking part in discussions and proposing training sessions are all ways of contributing to the vitality of the network.

    Mentoring: For more experienced nurses, mentoring young professionals is a valuable way of passing on knowledge and enriching the profession.

4. Overcoming challenges:

    Time: Although there are many benefits, active participation in a network requires time. It is essential to find a balance between professional responsibilities and involvement in these networks.

    Diversity of opinion: In any group, there will be differences of opinion. Active listening, mutual respect and a willingness to understand are essential to get the most out of these exchanges.

For the modern nurse, professional networks are much more than just a membership card. They represent an open door to better clinical practice, ongoing support and professional development. By becoming actively involved, nurses not only enrich their careers, but also contribute to the growth and vitality of the profession as a whole.

Continuing education and webinars

The dynamics of the medical world demand that skills and knowledge are constantly updated. Continuing education has become a cornerstone of the nursing profession, ensuring that caregivers have the tools and expertise they need to provide optimal care. In the digital age, webinars have become of paramount importance, offering unprecedented flexibility and access to education.

1. Continuing education: a professional imperative :
   - **Changing practices**: Techniques, drugs and technologies are evolving. Ongoing training enables nurses to keep abreast of these changes.
   - **Guaranteed quality of care**: Regular training ensures that patients receive care based on the latest evidence and recommendations.
   - **Professional development**: Training builds confidence and expertise, and can open doors to new specialisations or career opportunities.
2. Webinars: education just a click away :
   - **Flexibility**: Nurses often have busy and irregular schedules. Webinars can be followed live or on demand, depending on availability.
   - **Diversity of topics**: From wound management to psychology to technological innovations, there are webinars for every niche and interest.
   - **Interactivity**: Most webinars offer a question-and-answer session, allowing direct interaction with the experts.
3. How to maximise the effectiveness of webinars :
   - **Dedicated space**: Having a calm, distraction-free environment improves concentration and information retention.
   - **Active participation**: Asking questions, taking notes and engaging in post-webinar discussions reinforces learning.
   - **Putting it into practice**: After a webinar, it's a good idea to think about how you can incorporate this new learning into your day-to-day practice.

4. Finding the right resources :

> **Professional associations**: Many associations offer free or discounted webinars for their members.

> **Universities and institutions**: Many offer continuing education programmes, including webinars, for healthcare professionals.

> **Dedicated platforms**: There are specialised platforms that aggregate webinars from various fields, enabling nurses to choose sessions that meet their specific needs.

Continuing education is much more than a professional requirement: it's a demonstration of nurses' commitment to their profession and their patients. In a world where information is constantly at our fingertips, webinars represent a valuable opportunity for learning, growth and development.

Chapter 25:
HISTORY AND DEVELOPMENT
ALZHEIMER'S UNITS

Birth and necessity specialised units

As medicine and the understanding of disease progressed through the ages, the need for more targeted approaches to specific conditions became apparent. Specialist units, emerging as a response to this need, have transformed the way care is delivered, particularly for complex conditions such as Alzheimer's.

1. The evolution of patient care :
Over the decades, hospitals and care centres have evolved from generalist structures to entities where care is increasingly specialised. This has proved particularly beneficial for diseases requiring special attention, resources and skills.

2. Awareness of the complexity of Alzheimer's :
Alzheimer's disease, with its insidious progression and multiple facets, requires holistic care. It has become clear that care for these patients goes far beyond medical treatment, encompassing psychosocial, behavioural and environmental aspects.

3. **Birth of specialised units :**
In response to these challenges, specialised units began to emerge. These units, often integrated into long-term care facilities, were specifically designed to meet the unique needs of Alzheimer's patients.

4. The benefits of specialist care :

   Adapted environment: Specialised units are designed to take account of patients' cognitive and physical challenges, reducing risks such as falls or running away.

Specially trained teams: Staff in these units are trained to understand and respond to the behavioural manifestations often encountered in Alzheimer's patients.

Multidisciplinary approach: These units bring together a diverse team - doctors, nurses, occupational therapists, psychologists, etc. - to provide comprehensive care. - to provide comprehensive care.

Support for families: Recognising the emotional burden that illness can place on loved ones, these units often offer specific resources and support for families.

5. The future of specialist units :

With the growing prevalence of Alzheimer's disease and related disorders, the need for these specialist units will only increase. It is likely that the future will see an expansion of these units, as well as the emergence of new care modalities, technologies and innovative therapies.

The creation of specialised Alzheimer's units symbolises a major development in patient care. They embody recognition of the complexity of the disease and a commitment to a truly patient-centred approach to care.

Changes in practices and therapies

A look at the history of Alzheimer's care reveals a radical transformation in therapeutic approaches. The way in which we perceive, understand and treat this disease has evolved in leaps and bounds, reflecting medical advances, socio-cultural changes and a deepening of scientific knowledge.

1. Initial understanding :

In the early days of medical recognition of Alzheimer's disease, the condition was often misunderstood, confused with normal ageing or other psychiatric conditions. Interventions were largely non-specific, focused on patient comfort rather than a deep understanding of the disease.

2. Emergence of pharmacological therapies :

As research progressed, the first drugs specifically designed to treat Alzheimer's symptoms appeared. Although they do not offer a cure, they have marked a turning point in helping to manage certain symptoms and improve quality of life.

3. The rise of non-pharmacological therapies :

Alongside pharmacotherapy, a growing awareness of the importance of non-pharmacological interventions has emerged. Therapies such as music therapy, art therapy and cognitive stimulation therapy have begun to be integrated into care plans, underlining the importance of a holistic approach.

4. A patient-centred approach :

Over time, care has evolved to focus on the person rather than the disease. Rather than focusing solely on deficits, the approach has become more focused on the patient's residual strengths, seeking to maximise quality of life and independence.

5. Integrating technology :

The modern era has seen the increasing integration of technology into Alzheimer's patient care. From monitoring to cognitive stimulation and communication tools, technology has become a valuable ally for carers and patients alike.

<u>6. Towards a promising future :</u>
As research into Alzheimer's disease progresses, new therapies - whether pharmacological, technological or behavioural - continue to emerge. The trend is towards innovation, personalised care and interdisciplinary collaboration.

The development of practices and therapies for the treatment of Alzheimer's disease reflects a trajectory of learning, adaptation and innovation. It testifies to the medical world's ongoing commitment to improving the lives of patients and their families in the face of a complex and challenging disease.

Alzheimer's units
in different countries and cultures

Around the world, the way in which Alzheimer's disease is perceived, understood and treated varies considerably according to culture, healthcare systems and available resources. The existence and nature of dedicated Alzheimer's units are also influenced by these factors. Let's take a look at how different countries and cultures approach these specific units.

1. Western Europe :

France: Long-term care units (USLD) and establishments for dependent elderly people (EHPAD) may have specialised sections for Alzheimer's patients. These units are generally well-equipped and follow national guidelines for care.

Germany: Germany has a robust home care structure. However, there are also retirement homes and specialist facilities for patients suffering from dementia and Alzheimer's.

2. North America :
    United States: Memory Care Units are facilities specially designed for people with Alzheimer's or related dementias. They offer a secure environment with a focus on cognitive stimulation.
    Canada: Similar to the United States, Canada has specialist care centres for Alzheimer's patients with a holistic approach, including alternative therapies.

3. Asia :
    Japan: With a growing ageing population, Japan has set up "Group Homes", small-scale residences for Alzheimer's patients, offering personalised care in a family setting.
    India: Institutional care is less common. The family plays a central role in care. However, growing awareness of the disease is leading to the creation of specialist centres in major cities.

4. Africa :
    Awareness of Alzheimer's disease is growing, but resources and infrastructure for specialist units are lacking in many countries. Care is mainly provided by the family, with help from the community.

5. Latin America :
    In countries such as Brazil and Argentina, there are retirement homes with specialised sections for Alzheimer's patients. However, in many countries, the family remains the main provider of care.

6. Oceania :
    Australia: There are specialist units for Alzheimer's patients, often located within retirement homes or care facilities for the elderly. They focus on community involvement and cognitive stimulation.

The existence and operation of Alzheimer's units around the world reflect the diversity of cultural and systemic approaches to the disease. However, whatever the differences, the universal aim remains to provide quality care, ensure dignity and improve patients' quality of life.

Chapter 26:
DESIGN AND LAYOUT ALZHEIMER'S UNITS

Fundamental planning principles for Alzheimer's patients

Designing spaces for Alzheimer's patients requires an approach that is both sensitive and practical. These people are often disorientated, have memory problems and can be easily stressed by unfamiliar or complicated surroundings. Here is a fluid exploration of the key principles to consider when designing spaces for these patients.

When designing a unit or home for people with Alzheimer's, it's not just about creating a safe space; it's just as crucial to create an environment that supports their emotional, physical and cognitive well-being.

Alzheimer's patients need a space that, while familiar, is structured to minimise confusion and encourage independence. A floor with contrasting colours, for example, can help define the space and guide residents from one room to another. Winding corridors, on the other hand, can create confusion. Straight, well-lit corridors are a better option.

Lighting plays a crucial role. Plenty of natural light can help regulate circadian rhythms, reducing symptoms of 'twilight syndrome', where patients can become more agitated in the late afternoon. In addition, good lighting reduces the risk of falls, a common problem among Alzheimer's patients.

Another aspect to consider is sensory stimulation. Spaces that are too noisy or chaotic can be overwhelming. Nevertheless, a certain level of stimulation is beneficial. Therapeutic gardens, for example, can provide an oasis of calm. These gardens, with their fragrant flowers, chirping birds and winding paths, can be a source of comfort and soothing. They also encourage physical activity and a connection with nature, both of which are essential to the well-being of any individual.

And let's not forget the importance of personalisation. Every patient has their own story, their own tastes and their own experiences. Having areas where they can display personal photos or familiar objects can help create a sense of belonging and recognition.

Finally, safety is paramount. Water points, kitchens and even nooks and crannies can present dangers. So designing spaces where patients can move around freely, yet safely, is a delicate balance to strike.

Thoughtful design for Alzheimer's patients goes far beyond simple safety. It's about creating an environment where residents can not only live, but thrive, despite the challenges posed by the disease.

Importance of safety and surveillance

Safety and surveillance are central to the care of Alzheimer's patients. Because of the cognitive challenges posed by the disease, these individuals are particularly vulnerable to potential dangers in their environment, making it all the more crucial to put in place appropriate measures. The challenges of this safety go beyond mere physical protection; it also involves preserving the patient's dignity and autonomy while ensuring his or her safety.

Alzheimer's disease, by its very nature, is progressive. The early stages may manifest themselves as simple forgetfulness, but as the disease progresses, problems with disorientation, judgement and perception become more apparent. This evolution makes monitoring and safety essential at various levels.

One of the major risks for Alzheimer's patients is wandering. A patient may forget where they are or where they want to go, leading to potentially dangerous wandering. In these moments of confusion, the risk of falling, being injured or getting lost is increased. Monitoring systems, such as cameras or door alarms, can help care staff to intervene quickly if necessary.

At the same time, a delicate balance must be struck between surveillance and respect for the patient's privacy. While safety is paramount, it is also essential to preserve the patient's dignity and autonomy. Less intrusive solutions, such as motion sensors or identification bracelets, can be used to ensure effective surveillance while minimising intrusion.

The risks are not limited to ambulation. Patients can sometimes forget how to use everyday objects, such as household appliances, which can pose risks of fire or injury. Specific arrangements, such as deactivating certain appliances or using adapted equipment, can prevent such incidents.

Safety and monitoring are also crucial when administering medicines. Errors in dosage or taking medicines that have not been prescribed can have serious consequences. Electronic pillboxes or automated dispensing systems can help ensure that medicines are taken correctly.

Ensuring the safety of Alzheimer's patients is a multi-dimensional responsibility that requires a combination of technology, appropriate accommodation and careful monitoring. However, at the heart of all these measures is a fundamental principle: respect and kindness towards the patient, who, despite the challenges posed by his or her illness, deserves a life full of dignity, respect and quality.

Innovation and future trends in the design of the units

Advances in knowledge about Alzheimer's disease and the specific needs of patients have led to significant advances in the design of specialist units. Design innovation aims not only to ensure patients' safety, but also to create an environment that supports their emotional, social and physical well-being. Future trends reflect a patient-centred approach, seeking to replicate a familiar environment while incorporating the latest technologies.

At the heart of any good design for an Alzheimer's unit is the desire to recreate a space that feels as much like home as possible. Indeed, a familiar environment can help reduce the anxiety and confusion often felt by patients. This means smaller living spaces, similar to flats or houses, rather than long hospital corridors.

Another key element in modern design is natural light. Studies have shown that exposure to natural light can help regulate patients' circadian rhythms, reducing symptoms of the 'twilight syndrome' commonly seen in Alzheimer's sufferers. The new designs therefore incorporate large windows, skylights and interior gardens.

Talking of gardens, nature is playing an increasingly central role in the design of Alzheimer's units. Therapeutic gardens, which are secure and easily accessible, provide a space where patients can walk, garden or simply enjoy the outdoors. These green spaces not only serve as places to relax, but also provide sensory stimulation, which is essential for patients' well-being.

Technological innovation also plays a major role in current trends. Advanced surveillance systems, using motion sensors, smart cameras or even geolocation technologies, are being integrated to guarantee safety without being intrusive. In addition, technological solutions such as virtual reality or digital music therapies are being explored to offer innovative therapeutic interventions.

One of the most promising trends is the co-creative design approach, where patients, their families and carers work closely with architects and designers to create spaces that best meet the unique needs of each individual.

Finally, as research progresses, it is likely that we will see an increase in the personalisation of spaces. This could mean rooms that can be adapted to the patient's personal tastes, or communal spaces that can be modified to suit the day's activities.

The convergence of technology, research and deep empathy for Alzheimer's patients is shaping a future where specialist units are not only places of care, but also places of life, joy and dignity.

Chapter 27:
TECHNOLOGY AND INNOVATION

Technological tools
for assessment and monitoring

In the digital age, the use of technological tools to assess and monitor Alzheimer's patients has gained ground. These innovations aim not only to improve the quality of care, but also to facilitate the work of healthcare professionals and provide valuable information for families and carers. These tools play a crucial role in personalising care and predicting the progression of the disease.

One of the main advances is the use of wearables, such as smartwatches and wristbands, which can track a patient's movements, heart rate and sleep. These devices can detect changes in normal routines, such as increased restlessness at night, which could indicate disease progression or the presence of an underlying problem.

Mobile applications have also proved useful. There are now applications designed to test memory, attention and other cognitive functions. These regular assessments can help detect early declines, enabling earlier intervention. In addition, some applications provide reminders for medication, suggestions for adapted activities, and simplified means of communication for patients.

Online platforms dedicated to telemedicine and telemonitoring allow healthcare professionals to assess patients remotely, monitor disease progression and advise families without the need for frequent clinic visits. This approach is particularly beneficial for patients living in remote areas or who have difficulty travelling.

Virtual reality is another emerging technology in the Alzheimer's field. It can be used to create stimulating environments for patients, helping to slow cognitive decline. It also offers opportunities for assessment, by placing patients in a variety of situations and observing their reactions.

Artificial intelligence and machine learning systems are also at the forefront of Alzheimer's research. They analyse huge datasets to identify patterns or early indicators of the disease that might go unnoticed by the human eye.

Finally, advanced imaging tools, such as PET scanners and new-generation MRIs, allow more precise visualisation of changes in the brain. This gives doctors a better understanding of the progression of the disease and its impact on brain structure.

Technological tools for assessing and monitoring Alzheimer's patients are constantly evolving, promising to revolutionise the way we understand, treat and support those affected by this devastating disease.

Technologies to improve patients' quality of life

The impact of technology on the medical field is undeniable, and its influence on the care of Alzheimer's patients is no exception. These innovations, whether subtle or revolutionary, have the potential to improve patients' quality of life by offering them greater independence, security and the means to remain engaged with their environment.

1. Tracking and alert devices: GPS watches and other wearables can quickly locate a patient who may be lost, reducing the risks associated with disorientation.

2. Reminder applications: Applications specifically designed for Alzheimer's patients can help remind them of daily tasks, medical appointments and medication schedules, thereby promoting greater independence.

3. Interactive platforms: Tablets and dedicated applications can offer memory games, puzzles and other activities that stimulate the brain and keep patients engaged.

4. Virtual reality assisted therapies: Virtual reality can allow patients to visit places from their past, experience soothing environments, or even interact in social scenarios, providing a source of comfort and cognitive stimulation.

5. Voice recognition systems: These systems, such as Amazon Echo or Google Home, can help patients carry out everyday tasks, obtain information, or simply play music, all by voice commands.

6. Light therapy technology: Studies suggest that exposure to certain lights can improve sleep and reduce agitation in Alzheimer's patients. Light therapy lamps may therefore play a role in regulating circadian rhythms.

7. Enhanced communication: Special applications can make communication easier for those who have difficulty finding words, using images, pictograms and other visuals.

8. Robotics: Although it may seem futuristic, robots such as Paro, a robotic cuddly toy in the shape of a seal, have been designed to offer comfort and reduce patient anxiety.

9. Home assistance systems: These systems can detect falls, unusual movements or an absence of activity over an extended period, sending alerts to carers or family members.

10. Intelligent hearing aids : These devices do more than just amplify sound. They can filter out background noise and focus on conversations, which is particularly useful in noisy environments.

In conclusion, as technology continues to evolve at a rapid pace, it is essential to recognise its potential to improve the lives of Alzheimer's patients. These tools can help bridge the gap between the needs of patients and the capabilities of carers, while offering moments of joy, comfort and independence.

Limits and challenges technological integration

The advent of technology in healthcare has undoubtedly brought many benefits, particularly for Alzheimer's patients. However, its integration also presents challenges and limitations that it is crucial to recognise and understand.

1. Resistance to adoption: Technology can be intimidating, especially for older people who are not used to it. This can lead to hesitation or outright rejection, making it difficult to implement technological solutions.

2. High costs: Technological devices and specialist software can be expensive, which may limit their accessibility to all patients, particularly those who are economically disadvantaged.

3. Confidentiality and security: Monitoring systems and other connected devices raise concerns about the confidentiality of patient data and the security of this information against cyber-attacks.

4. Complexity and training: Implementing new technologies often requires training for care staff, which can be a constraint on time and resources.

5. Risk of dependency: Over-reliance on technology can potentially reduce human interaction, which is fundamental to the emotional and social health of Alzheimer's patients.

6. Unsuitability: Not all technologies are suitable for every stage of the disease. What works for a patient at the beginning of the disease may not be effective at a more advanced stage.

7. Rapid obsolescence: With the rapid pace of technological progress, devices can quickly become obsolete, requiring frequent upgrades and additional investment.

8. Data integrity : Technological tools can sometimes malfunction, giving inaccurate readings or data that could mislead carers.

9. Sensory overload: For some patients, excessive use of technology can lead to information overload or overstimulation, which can be uncomfortable or stressful.

10. Physiological limitations: Technologies such as virtual reality may not be suitable for all patients, especially if they cause dizziness, nausea or other adverse effects.

Although technology offers great potential for improving the quality of life of Alzheimer's patients, it must be integrated with care and sensitivity. Carers and healthcare professionals need to be aware of these challenges to ensure thoughtful, balanced and patient-centred implementation.

Chapter 28:
THE CHALLENGES OF THE NIGHT IN AN ALZHEIMER'S UNIT

Particularities of night work

Working at night in specialised Alzheimer's units brings its own challenges and particularities. Being a healthcare professional working during these hours can be a singular experience, requiring specific skills, sensitivity and adaptability.

1. Twilight syndrome: Many Alzheimer's patients may experience increased agitation or confusion during the twilight or night hours, known as "twilight syndrome". This requires extra vigilance on the part of night staff.

2. Quiet environment: At night, units tend to be quieter, with fewer external stimuli, which can be beneficial for some patients but disruptive for others.

3. Monitoring wandering: Some patients may have a tendency to wander during the night. Night staff must ensure that these patients do not injure themselves and remain safe.

4. Circadian rhythm: Disruption of the sleep-wake cycle is common in Alzheimer's patients. Night staff must be trained to manage patients who are awake and active for long periods at night.

5. Limited intervention: At night, there are generally fewer staff available, which means that carers need to be well trained to manage a variety of situations with limited resources.

6. Appropriate activities: Some patients may need activities to keep them occupied at night. These activities should be soothing and non-stimulating to avoid aggravating the agitation.

7. Light management: Lighting is crucial. Soft, soothing light can help prevent agitation, while appropriate lighting can help reset patients' body clocks.

8. Noise and sound : Noise control is essential at night. Soothing sounds or soft music can help calm an agitated patient, while loud or sudden noises can be disruptive.

9. Emotional support: Patients may feel more vulnerable or anxious at night. Staff must be trained to provide appropriate emotional support.

10. Staff self-care: Working nights can have an impact on staff health and well-being. Implementing self-care strategies, such as regular breaks and good hydration, is crucial.

Working at night in an Alzheimer's unit requires a specific, patient-centred approach, adapted to the unique challenges that these hours bring. The carers working during these periods play an essential role in the care and well-being of patients.

Managing sleep disorders

Sleep disorders are common in Alzheimer's patients. These disorders can manifest themselves in a variety of ways, ranging from insomnia to excessive sleepiness and changes in circadian rhythm. Not only can these sleep disturbances exacerbate the cognitive, behavioural and psychological symptoms of dementia, they can also have a negative impact on the patient's quality of life and increase the workload of carers.

1. Understanding the problem: The first step towards managing sleep disorders is to recognise their presence.

This may require careful monitoring of the patient's sleep patterns, sometimes using sleep tracking devices.

2. Maintain a regular routine: Helping patients to establish and maintain a regular daily routine can help regulate the sleep-wake cycle. This includes going to bed and waking up at set times.

3. Light therapy: Exposure to natural light during the day, especially in the morning, can help to reset the patient's biological clock. If this is not possible, light therapy lamps can be used.

4. Comfortable sleeping environment: Make sure the bedroom is conducive to sleep - dark, quiet and cool. Avoid screens and bright lights before bedtime.

5. Physical activity: Encouraging patients to exercise during the day, even just walking, can help them sleep better at night.

6. Managing caffeine and diet: Limit caffeine intake, especially in the late afternoon and evening, and avoid heavy meals before bedtime.

7. Medication: Some medicines can disrupt sleep. It is therefore essential to regularly review the patient's medication with a healthcare professional. In some cases, specific medicines may be prescribed to help regulate sleep.

8. Relaxation techniques: Methods such as meditation, deep breathing and music therapy can help to relax the patient before bedtime.

9. Managing nocturnal symptoms: If the patient wakes up at night because of agitation or anxiety, gentle, soothing interventions, rather than abrupt reactions, can help to reassure them and get them back to sleep.

10. Support for carers: Educating and supporting carers is crucial. Their sleep patterns can also be disrupted, and giving them tools and strategies to manage sleep disorders can benefit both them and the patient.

Treating sleep disorders in Alzheimer's patients requires an individualised and holistic approach. By working closely with carers and combining non-medicinal interventions with, if necessary, medicinal treatments, it is possible to improve sleep quality and, consequently, patients' quality of life.

Protocols and procedures for night shifts

Night teams in Alzheimer's units play a crucial role in ensuring the safety, comfort and well-being of patients. The nature of Alzheimer's disease can lead to unpredictable nocturnal behaviour, requiring special attention and adapted protocols. Here is an overview of the protocols and procedures for these teams:

1. Handover between teams :
Clear and comprehensive communication between the day and night teams is essential. It enables all relevant information to be passed on about the condition of patients, incidents that have occurred during the day and any special features to be monitored.

2. Regular checks :
Patients must be checked regularly throughout the night to ensure their well-being, but also to detect and intervene in the event of unexpected behaviour.

3. Managing night-time awakenings :
Specific protocols must be in place to manage night-time awakenings, whether due to agitation, confusion or other symptoms. It is crucial to approach patients with calm and empathy.

4. Falls prevention :
Preventive measures, such as the use of bed rails, night lighting and non-slip mats, can help prevent falls. Careful supervision is also essential, especially for patients who may get up frequently during the night.

5. Medication :
Some patients may require medication during the night. Night nurses need to know the timing of these drugs and their potential effects. Good stock management and accurate documentation are also essential.

6. Noise management :
Noise should be kept to a minimum to promote a peaceful sleeping environment. This includes minimising loud talking, using quiet equipment and respecting sleeping areas.

7. Emergency situations :
Night teams need to be well trained to deal with emergencies, whether medical complications, aggressive behaviour or other crises.

8. Documentation :
All observations, incidents and interventions must be carefully documented to ensure continuity of care and to inform the morning team of the events of the night.

9. Mutual support :
Night work can be isolating, so staff should be encouraged to support each other. Close collaboration and open communication between team members are essential.

10. Further training :
Night staff should have the same opportunities for ongoing training as day staff, particularly in the latest practices and research relating to Alzheimer's disease.

Ensuring the well-being of Alzheimer's patients at night requires dedication, expertise and a tailored approach. With clear protocols in place and ongoing training and support, night teams can provide exceptional care for this vulnerable population.

Chapter 29:
GLOBAL APPROACHES
AND INTEGRATIVE

The importance of
a holistic approach to care

The treatment of Alzheimer's disease, like that of many other chronic conditions, cannot be limited to a reductive and symptomatic vision. To be truly effective and respectful of the individual, it must adopt a holistic perspective. But what exactly does this mean, and why is it so crucial?

A holistic approach to care takes into account the whole person, i.e. not only their physiological needs, but also their psychological, social, spiritual and emotional needs. It recognises that each individual is unique and that the symptoms of an illness can affect different facets of their lives.

1. Recognising the person behind the disease :
Every Alzheimer's patient has a story, desires, fears, loves and dislikes. Holistic care seeks to honour this individuality, to recognise the intrinsic value and dignity of each person, regardless of the stage of their illness.

2. Personalised care:
By taking into account each patient's history, preferences and needs, carers can tailor interventions and treatments to be as beneficial and meaningful as possible.

3. Integrating emotional and spiritual dimensions :
The progression of Alzheimer's disease can raise existential questions for both patients and their loved ones. Holistic care includes spiritual and emotional support as an essential element of overall well-being.

4. The importance of relationships :
Maintaining meaningful relationships is fundamental to human wellbeing. A holistic approach values and supports relationships between the patient, family, friends and carers, recognising that each plays a vital role in the patient's support network.

5. Integrating complementary therapies :
In addition to traditional medical and pharmacological interventions, a holistic vision can integrate complementary therapies such as music therapy, aromatherapy, art therapy and other modalities to support overall wellbeing.

6. Support for carers:
A holistic approach also recognises the needs of carers, who can experience significant emotional, physical and psychological stress. Providing them with support, training and resources is crucial to ensuring quality care.

A holistic approach to care aims to ensure the respect, dignity and well-being of people with Alzheimer's disease. It seeks to look beyond the symptoms and respond to the complex and interdependent needs of each individual, offering more comprehensive and humane care.

Integration of practices traditional and alternative

Alzheimer's disease, with its intrinsic complexity, has prompted many carers, researchers and families to broaden the spectrum of therapeutic interventions available. In addition to conventional medical approaches, many traditional and alternative practices have shown promising potential for supporting people with this degenerative condition.

Historically, traditional medicine has been the backbone of healthcare systems in many cultures around the world.

These approaches, often inherited from centuries of wisdom and practice, offer different perspectives and methods from those of Western medicine. In addition, alternative therapies, although more recent, often seek to fill the gaps left by conventional interventions.

1. Traditional Chinese Medicine (TCM):
Studies have shown that certain herbs used in TCM, such as Ginkgo biloba, may offer cognitive benefits for Alzheimer's patients, although the evidence remains mixed.

2. Ayurveda:
This traditional Indian medicine uses a combination of herbs, diet and physical practices (such as yoga) to balance the body and mind. Ashwagandha, for example, is an herb often recommended to support cognitive health.

3. Aromatherapy:
Essential oils such as lavender or rosemary are used to calm anxiety or stimulate memory, respectively. Although not curative, they can improve quality of life.

4. Nutritional approaches :
Diets such as the Mediterranean diet or the MIND diet, rich in antioxidants and omega-3 fatty acids, have been associated with better cognitive health.

5. Energy therapies:
Techniques such as Reiki or Qi Gong seek to balance the body's vital energy and can help manage stress and anxiety.

6. Massage and therapeutic touch :
These techniques can help reduce anxiety, improve mood and improve circulation.

Integrating these traditional and alternative therapies requires a cautious approach. It is essential to ensure that any intervention is safe and does not contradict ongoing medical treatment. In addition, it is crucial to recognise that, although these methods can offer valuable support, they do not replace conventional medical interventions but complement them.

An open dialogue between patients, families, carers and healthcare professionals is therefore essential for successful integration. With a holistic vision of care, embracing both conventional and alternative practices, we can offer a wider range of options to improve the quality of life of people with Alzheimer's disease.

Collaborate
with non-conventional practitioners

In the complex landscape of Alzheimer's disease care, there is a range of therapists and practitioners who offer unconventional interventions. These interventions, which range from traditional medicine to complementary and alternative therapies, can provide an extra dimension of support for patients and their families.

One of the first steps in working with non-conventional practitioners is the mutual recognition of the unique role each plays in the overall wellbeing of the patient. Where conventional medicine may focus on symptoms, disease progression and medication, non-conventional practitioners can offer methods that aim to improve quality of life, manage stress and support emotional and spiritual well-being.

1. Establish open communication :
Regular and transparent dialogue between conventional and non-conventional practitioners ensures that all care is coordinated and focused on the patient's best interests. It can also help to identify any potential interactions or contraindications between different interventions.

2. Mutual education :
Understanding the basics of different treatment modalities allows for smoother collaboration. Workshops or seminars can be organised so that practitioners from both sides can learn from each other.

3. Integrated care planning :
Creating a care plan that includes both conventional and non-conventional interventions provides a holistic approach. This may include medication, aromatherapy, massage, acupuncture or other therapies.

4. Ensuring safety:
While recognising the value of unconventional interventions, it is crucial to ensure that they are safe for the patient. Verification of qualifications, monitoring of potential drug interactions and consideration of the patient's specific needs are essential.

5. Recognise and respect patients' and families' choices :
Decisions about care should always be made with the patient and their family. Shared decision-making ensures that care reflects the patient's values, beliefs and preferences.

The main aim of collaborating with unconventional practitioners is to offer Alzheimer's patients the fullest and most caring spectrum of care possible. By integrating interventions that address the physical, emotional and spiritual, we can hope to offer an improved quality of life to those navigating the challenges of this degenerative disease.

Chapter 30:
MANAGEMENT PAIN AND DISCOMFORT

Pain assessment
in non-communicative patients

Assessing pain in non-communicative patients, such as those with advanced Alzheimer's disease or other neurodegenerative conditions, is a major challenge for healthcare professionals. These patients often cannot verbally express their feelings or discomfort. However, untreated pain can lead to complications and significantly reduce quality of life. Here's how to make an effective assessment in these circumstances:

1. Observe behavioural changes :
Non-communicative patients may express their pain through non-verbal behaviour. This may include grimacing, crying, agitation, isolation or even aggressive behaviour. Particular attention should be paid to these signs, especially after a procedure or movement likely to cause pain.

2. Look for physiological signs:
Changes in vital signs, such as increased heart rate, blood pressure or breathing, can be indicators of pain. Similarly, sweating or redness can be signals.

3. Use specific assessment scales :
There are pain assessment scales designed specifically for non-communicative patients. Scales such as DOLOPLUS-2 or PAINAD can be useful for quantifying and monitoring pain in these patients on the basis of various behavioural indicators.

4. Assess regularly:
Pain should be assessed regularly, particularly after

procedures or treatments that could increase discomfort. Ongoing assessment allows interventions to be adjusted accordingly.

5. Ask those close to you:
Family and carers can often recognise subtle signs of pain that medical staff may miss. They know the patient and can spot changes in habits or behaviour.

6. Targeted physical examination :
A physical examination can help locate the source of the pain. For example, an inflamed area, injury or infection may be identified during the examination.

7. Opt for multimodal interventions:
Once pain has been identified, it should be treated using a combination of approaches, which may include medication, physical therapies and non-pharmacological interventions such as music or therapeutic touch.

Recognising and treating pain in non-communicative patients is essential to improving their quality of life. Although this is a challenge, with careful observation and regular assessment, healthcare professionals can respond effectively to the needs of these vulnerable patients.

Non-pharmacological techniques pain management

Pain management is a central part of patient care, and although drugs play a crucial role in this process, non-pharmacological approaches offer important alternatives, particularly for those who may be sensitive to the side effects of drugs or who are looking to supplement their treatment regime. Here is an exploration of some of these techniques:

1. Physical therapy :
   - **Physiotherapy:** This can help to strengthen muscles, increase flexibility and improve mobility, which in turn can reduce pain, particularly that associated with musculoskeletal conditions.
   - **Hydrotherapy:** The use of water, hot or cold, to relieve pain. For example, a hot bath can relax muscles and increase blood circulation.
2. Body-mind therapies :
   - **Meditation and mindfulness:** These practices help to refocus the mind and can reduce the perception of pain.
   - **Biofeedback:** A technique in which you learn to control physiological functions in order to reduce pain.
   - **Guided relaxation:** Using visualisation or progressive muscle relaxation to reduce tension and pain.
3. Manual therapies :
   - **Massage therapy:** Massage can relax muscles, increase blood circulation and improve general well-being.
   - **Chiropractic:** Chiropractic adjustments can help to align the spine, thereby reducing pain.
   - **Osteopathy:** A holistic approach that focuses on treating the whole body to relieve pain.
4. Energy approaches :
   - **Acupuncture:** This ancient Chinese practice uses fine needles inserted at specific points on the body to reduce pain.
   - **Reiki: An** energy healing method that can help balance the body's energies and reduce pain.
5. Heating and cooling applications :
   - Heat can relax and soothe muscles while increasing blood flow, while cold can reduce inflammation and numb the painful area.

6. Transcutaneous electrical stimulation (TENS) :
   * A small machine sends electrical impulses to the skin to reduce the perception of pain.
7. Art therapies :
   * Music therapy, art therapy and dance therapy can help to divert attention from the pain and manage it emotionally.
8. Education and self-management :
   * Learning about pain, its causes and how to manage it can give patients the tools they need to take better control of their condition.

It is important to remember that pain is a subjective experience, and what works for one patient may not work for another. An individualised and holistic approach, combining pharmacological and non-pharmacological methods, offers the best chance of success in pain management.

The importance of interpretation non-verbal signals

In the world of care and well-being, particularly for people with neurodegenerative diseases such as Alzheimer's, the importance of interpreting non-verbal cues cannot be underestimated. Here's why:

* **Primary expression of needs and emotions:** In patients who have difficulty communicating verbally, gestures, facial expressions and posture often become the primary means of expressing needs, discomfort, pain or emotions.
* **Early identification of problems:** For example, a patient who grimaces may be in pain. A patient who withdraws could indicate anxiety or fear.

- **Establishing a relationship of trust:** When carers pay attention to and respond appropriately to non-verbal cues, this can build trust and comfort between carer and patient.
- **Preventing conflict situations:** By recognising signs of agitation or distress early on, it is possible to intervene before the patient becomes aggressive or extremely stressed.
- **Facilitating communication:** For people with problems speaking or formulating thoughts, correctly interpreting non-verbal signals can greatly facilitate understanding and exchange.
- **Cultural understanding:** Certain non-verbal signals can have different meanings in different cultures. Being sensitive and informed about this can help avoid misunderstandings.
- **Evaluating the effectiveness of care:** Patients' non-verbal reactions can provide clues as to the effectiveness of a treatment or intervention. For example, a patient may relax after receiving pain medication, signalling a reduction in pain.
- **Supporting patient dignity:** By paying attention to non-verbal cues, carers recognise and validate the patient's experience, which can support the patient's sense of dignity and self-esteem.

While words are powerful vectors of communication, non-verbal signals offer a valuable window into the emotional, physical and mental state of patients, particularly those who may not be able to express themselves fully through speech. Careful interpretation of these signals is essential to providing compassionate, effective and individualised care.

Chapter 31:
THE IMPACT OF CULTURE AND DIVERSITY IN CARE

Understanding cultural variations in the perception of illness

The perception of illness, and in particular diseases such as Alzheimer's, varies considerably from one culture to another. These cultural differences influence not only how the disease is perceived and understood, but also how it is managed and treated.

- **Aetiology and interpretation:** In some cultures, Alzheimer's disease and other forms of dementia are seen not as neurodegenerative diseases, but as a normal part of ageing, or even as a curse, a spell or the result of past actions.
- **Stigma:** In some environments, the diagnosis of Alzheimer's disease can lead to significant stigma, which can discourage families from seeking help or even admitting that the disease exists. This stigma can also affect the person with the disease, leading to isolation and a lack of access to appropriate care.
- **Family roles and responsibilities:** Cultural expectations can influence how care responsibilities are divided within the family. For example, in some cultures the eldest son or daughter may be expected to take primary responsibility for care, while in others this responsibility may be shared more widely.
- **Attitudes towards professional care:** In some cultures, care of the elderly or sick at home by the family is the norm, and the idea of entrusting a loved one to an institution is unthinkable. This contrasts

with other cultures where institutional or professional care may be more widely accepted.

- **Coping and support strategies:** Spiritual, religious and community resources play a crucial role in the way many cultures deal with illness. Prayer, ritual and ceremony can be important coping mechanisms.
- **Communication and expression:** The way in which symptoms are described, and the willingness to talk openly about them, can vary. In some cultures, emotional or behavioural symptoms may be emphasised, while in others, physical symptoms may be more commonly reported.
- **Medical and ethical decisions:** Attitudes towards informed consent, disclosure of diagnosis, end of life and advance directives are profoundly influenced by cultural factors.

Recognising and understanding these cultural variations is essential to providing effective and compassionate care. Healthcare professionals must be trained in cultural competence, in order to interact with patients and families in a way that is respectful and sensitive to their beliefs, values and preferences.

Adapting care by ethnic and religious diversity

At a time when globalisation is making our societies increasingly diverse, it is crucial to adapt care to take account of patients' different ethnic and religious backgrounds, particularly in sensitive areas such as Alzheimer's care.

- **Cultural knowledge:** The first step in adapting care is to acquire knowledge of the main beliefs, practices and values associated with different ethnic groups and religions. This knowledge enables healthcare professionals to better understand the context in which patients perceive and experience their illness.

- **Cultural competence training: It's** not enough to know about different cultures, you also need to know how to integrate this knowledge into everyday clinical practice. This helps to avoid misunderstandings, improve communication and provide appropriate care.

- **Individual assessment:** Even within the same ethnic group or religion, beliefs and practices can vary from one person to another. It is therefore crucial to ask open-ended questions to understand the specific needs of each patient.

- **Respect for rites and rituals:** Certain practices or rituals may be of great importance to patients and their families. For example, prayer rites at specific times, dietary restrictions or end-of-life rituals.

- **Language and communication:** Language barriers can be a major obstacle. The use of interpreters or translation technologies can help to ensure that the patient and their family fully understand medical information and recommendations.

- **Including the family:** In many cultures, the family plays a central role in medical decision-making. It is therefore essential to include them in discussions and care plans.

- **Adapting interventions :** Therapeutic interventions, whether medical, psychosocial or other, need to be adapted to take account of the patient's beliefs and values. This may include modifying therapeutic approaches or seeking alternatives that are culturally appropriate.

- **Collaboration with community leaders:** In certain situations, it may be beneficial to collaborate with religious or community leaders for advice or to facilitate communication and understanding between medical staff and the patient or family.

- **Culturally appropriate resources and materials:** Providing brochures, videos or other educational materials that reflect the patient's culture and language can greatly improve understanding and adherence to treatment.
- **Ongoing feedback:** It is important to encourage patients and their families to give feedback on the care they receive, in order to constantly adjust and improve culturally sensitive approaches.

Taking account of ethnic and religious diversity is not just a question of respect, it is also a way of improving the quality of care, building trust and ensuring that each patient receives the support most appropriate to their unique situation.

Training and awareness-raising to diversity for carers

In an ever-changing world, marked by globalisation and the mixing of cultures, it is becoming imperative for carers to acquire in-depth training and awareness of diversity. This approach, far from being a simple addition to their skills, is essential if they are to meet the changing needs of patients from a variety of backgrounds.

Diversity training is not limited to simple knowledge of different cultures or religions. It is deeply rooted in understanding the nuances, beliefs and behaviours that influence the way people perceive health, illness and medical care. It is a learning journey in which carers often find themselves challenging their own prejudices and stereotypes, in order to better understand and respect those they care for.

But why is this so crucial? The reason is simple: a better understanding of patients' cultural and ethnic backgrounds leads to smoother communication, better adherence to treatment and, ultimately, better care. Patients feel understood, respected and more willing to collaborate when they feel that their beliefs and values are taken into account.

Awareness-raising, on the other hand, goes beyond training. It involves an ongoing commitment to being aware of differences, keeping abreast of cultural developments and actively seeking out opportunities to learn. This can take the form of workshops, group discussions or even intercultural exchanges. Carers can also benefit from networking with healthcare professionals from other cultures, learning directly from authentic sources.

However, despite all their training and awareness, carers are also encouraged not to make hasty generalisations. Each individual is unique, and beliefs and behaviours can vary considerably even within the same culture or religion. It is therefore essential to adopt an individualised approach, asking open questions and listening actively.

The aim is to build bridges of mutual understanding and respect between carers and their patients. In a world where diversity is the norm rather than the exception, diversity training and awareness are not only desirable, they are absolutely necessary.

Chapter 32:
RESEARCH INTO ALZHEIMER'S PREVENTION

The latest findings on risk factors

Research into Alzheimer's disease is constantly evolving, with new discoveries regularly emerging to shed light on the causes and risk factors associated with this degenerative disease. Here is a fluid overview of recent discoveries concerning the risk factors for Alzheimer's disease:

Advances in Alzheimer's disease research in recent years have broadened our understanding of the risk factors associated with this devastating condition. While age, family history and genetics remain the predominant factors, new findings suggest that environment, lifestyle and other biological factors may also play a crucial role in the development of the disease.

Firstly, cardiovascular health is now widely recognised as being linked to brain health. High blood pressure, diabetes, obesity and smoking can all increase the risk of developing Alzheimer's disease. The reason for this? These conditions can compromise blood flow to the brain, affecting neurological processes.

In addition, studies have shown that sleep plays an essential role in the process of 'cleaning' the brain. Chronic sleep disturbance could prevent the brain from effectively eliminating beta-amyloid proteins, which accumulate and form plaques associated with Alzheimer's disease.

Environmental factors, such as exposure to certain toxins or pollutants, are also being studied. Some researchers are examining the link between exposure to heavy metals, such as aluminium, and the onset of the disease, although the results are still debated.

The intestinal microbiome, the complex ecosystem of bacteria living in our intestines, is also under the spotlight. Research suggests that an imbalance in these bacteria could have inflammatory consequences that have repercussions for the brain.

Finally, mental health could also be a factor. Depression, chronic stress or prolonged anxiety have been associated with an increased risk of dementia. While the causal link has not yet been clearly established, these conditions may aggravate symptoms or accelerate the progression of the disease.

It is essential to note that the presence of one or more of these risk factors does not guarantee the development of Alzheimer's disease. However, understanding them can pave the way for preventive interventions, earlier management and better prospects for those affected or at risk.

Diet, lifestyle and prevention

The relationship between diet, lifestyle and the prevention of Alzheimer's disease is an area of growing interest. Numerous studies have shown that a healthy lifestyle can not only reduce the risk of cardiovascular disease, diabetes and other conditions, but also have a positive impact on cognitive health. Find out how diet and lifestyle can play a role in preventing Alzheimer's disease.

The Mediterranean diet, rich in fruit, vegetables, olive oil, nuts, fish and whole grains, has been associated with a reduced risk of neurodegenerative diseases. This diet promotes the consumption of antioxidants and omega-3 fatty acids, which can protect the brain against oxidative damage and inflammation. Limiting consumption of red meat, processed foods and sugar can also help prevent the accumulation of beta-amyloid plaques, linked to Alzheimer's disease.

Regular physical activity is another essential pillar of prevention. Exercise improves blood flow to the brain, promotes neuroplasticity and can help prevent brain atrophy. Walking, swimming, yoga or any other form of activity that increases the heart rate can contribute to brain health.

Mental and social engagement is just as important. Reading, thinking games, lifelong learning and social interaction can strengthen the brain's resilience in the face of stress. Maintaining an active social network, participating in groups or clubs, and even simple activities such as chatting with friends can play a protective role against cognitive decline.

Sleep also plays a crucial role in prevention. During deep sleep, the brain 'cleans' waste products, including beta-amyloid proteins. So getting enough quality sleep can reduce the risk of these proteins accumulating.

Other lifestyle factors, such as stress management, meditation and relaxing activities, can also have a positive impact on cognitive health. Chronic stress releases cortisol, a hormone that can damage the brain in the long term.

Finally, moderating alcohol consumption, stopping smoking and regularly monitoring health parameters such as blood pressure, cholesterol and blood sugar levels can also contribute to prevention.

Although genetics play a role in Alzheimer's disease, healthy lifestyle choices can significantly reduce the risk or delay the onset of the disease. Adopting a holistic approach, integrating diet, exercise, mental and social engagement, can offer robust protection against cognitive decline.

Implications for nursing practice

Nursing practice is at the heart of healthcare, and recent discoveries concerning the prevention of Alzheimer's disease through diet and lifestyle have direct implications for nurses. Nurses play a central role in educating, supporting and implementing these preventive measures. Let's look at how these findings can be integrated into nursing practice:

- **Patient education**: Nurses can inform patients about the benefits of a healthy diet, particularly the Mediterranean diet, and the importance of regular exercise. This can be done during routine visits or through workshops and seminars.
- **Assessment of lifestyle habits**: During health checks, nurses can assess patients' eating habits, level of physical activity, sleep, stress and alcohol and tobacco consumption. This enables them to target areas for improvement.
- **Drawing up action plans**: On the basis of the assessment, nurses can help patients to draw up personalised action plans for adopting a healthier lifestyle.
- **Emotional and psychological support**: The prospect of developing Alzheimer's disease can be

frightening. Nurses can offer emotional support, listen to patients' concerns and refer them to appropriate resources or professionals if necessary.

- **Collaboration with other professionals**: Nurses can work with nutritionists, physiotherapists, psychologists and other professionals to provide comprehensive care. For example, if a patient has sleep problems, a referral to a sleep specialist could be beneficial.
- **Continuing education**: With constant advances in Alzheimer's research, it is crucial for nurses to stay up to date. Attending training courses, workshops and conferences can help them acquire new knowledge and skills.
- **Community health   promotion**: Beyond individual care, nurses can engage in community initiatives to promote healthy eating, physical activity and other aspects of a healthy lifestyle.
- **Documentation and research**: By recording the results of lifestyle interventions and participating in studies, nurses can contribute to the knowledge base on the effectiveness of interventions.
- **Advocacy**: Nurses, as patient advocates, can advocate for policies that support healthy environments, such as green spaces for exercise or access to nutritious food.

Nurses, thanks to their unique position in the healthcare system, have the potential to incorporate this knowledge of Alzheimer's prevention into their daily practices, thereby making a positive difference to the lives of many patients.

Chapter 33:
THE FUTURE OF CARE AND TREATMENT

Prospects and hopes in medical research

Medical research has always been the beacon guiding advances in healthcare. It builds on past discoveries, overcomes present challenges and illuminates future hopes for patients, carers and society as a whole. The current prospects and hopes for medical research are varied and touch on many areas. Here's an overview:

- **Genomic research**: With advances in the sequencing of the human genome, personalised medicine is becoming increasingly feasible. It is hoped that the identification of genetic mutations and biomarkers will be able to guide tailor-made treatments for diseases such as cancer, heart disease and neurodegenerative disorders.
- **Cellular therapies**: Stem cells, with their ability to transform into any type of cell in the body, offer enormous potential. Studies are underway to use stem cells to regenerate damaged tissue, such as after a heart attack, or to treat diseases such as diabetes.
- **Immunotherapy**: This is a revolutionary approach to treating cancer by 'educating' the immune system to recognise and attack cancer cells. Treatments such as checkpoint inhibitors and CAR-T cells have shown promising results.
- **CRISPR and gene-editing technologies**: The ability to 'correct' genetic mutations at source could revolutionise the treatment of rare genetic diseases.

- **Nanomedicine**: The use of nanoparticles to target drug delivery promises to reduce side effects and increase the effectiveness of treatments.
- **Microbiome research**: Our understanding of the importance of the billions of micro-organisms living in our bodies, particularly in the intestine, has exploded. This research could lead to new approaches to treating illnesses ranging from depression to inflammatory bowel disease.
- **Remote monitoring and intervention technologies**: With telemedicine and portable devices, remote monitoring and intervention are becoming possible, which could transform the way care is delivered, especially in remote areas.
- **Artificial intelligence (AI)**: AI and machine learning are being used more and more in diagnosis, the interpretation of medical images and even the prediction of epidemics.
- **Neuroscience**: Understanding the brain, with its myriad complexities, is a major area of research. Hopes are pinned on the treatment of diseases such as Alzheimer's, schizophrenia and depression.
- **Research into infectious diseases**: The COVID-19 pandemic served as a reminder of the importance of research into infectious diseases. Messenger RNA vaccines, which were developed in record time, are an example of innovation in this field.

Medical research is at an exciting crossroads, with many promising avenues open to it. While challenges remain, innovation, perseverance and global collaboration will continue to push the boundaries of what is medically possible.

The role of technology in the future of care

Technology, with its rapid evolution and ability to transform entire industries, is playing an increasingly central role in healthcare. Its capacity to facilitate, improve and revolutionise care is impressive. Here's how technology could play a key role in the future of healthcare:

- **Telemedicine and remote care**: Telemedicine has already demonstrated its potential during the COVID-19 pandemic, enabling patients to access consultations without leaving their homes. It also reduces geographical barriers, giving patients in rural or remote areas easier access to specialists.
- **Wearable devices and real-time monitoring**: Smartwatches, wristbands and other wearable devices allow real-time monitoring of parameters such as heart rate, blood pressure or blood sugar levels. This data can alert patients and healthcare professionals to potential problems before they become critical.
- **Artificial intelligence and diagnostics**: AI has the potential to rapidly and accurately analyse huge volumes of data, in particular to aid diagnosis, predict the risk of disease or even suggest treatments.
- **Robotics and surgery**: Robotic assistants can increase surgeons' precision, enable minimally invasive procedures and reduce recovery times for patients.
- **3D printing**: From the creation of made-to-measure prostheses to the manufacture of tissues and organs, 3D printing has the potential to revolutionise the way we approach healthcare.

- **Virtual and augmented reality**: Whether for training healthcare professionals, rehabilitating patients or managing pain, virtual and augmented reality offers innovative opportunities.
- **Genetic and personalised therapies**: Thanks to technological advances in genomic sequencing, we are moving towards personalised treatments based on individual genetics.
- **Interconnection and electronic medical records**: Fast, secure access to patients' medical records can make it easier to coordinate care and avoid medical errors.
- **Security and confidentiality**: With the increasing digitisation of healthcare data, technology also plays a crucial role in protecting this data against breaches and cyber-attacks.
- **Education and awareness**: Online platforms, applications and interactive tools can facilitate the ongoing training of healthcare professionals and the education of patients about their own conditions.

Technology promises to make healthcare more efficient, accessible and personalised. However, it must be deployed with care, taking into account ethical concerns, data security and equity of access. By putting patients at the heart of these innovations, we can look forward to a future where technology enriches the healthcare experience for all.

Vision on the evolution of the nursing profession in Alzheimer's units

The Alzheimer's nursing profession faces unique challenges, given the complex and progressive nature of Alzheimer's disease. This condition, combined with an ageing population in many countries, means that the demand for specialist care is likely to increase in the coming years. Here is a vision of the potential evolution of nursing in this field:

- **Increased specialisation**: Nurses working in Alzheimer's units may require more specialised training to effectively manage the behavioural and psychological symptoms of dementia.
- **Increasing use of technology**: As mentioned earlier, the integration of technology into the care of Alzheimer's patients will be essential. Whether for monitoring, engagement or training, nurses will need to be comfortable with these tools.
- **Holistic approach to care**: Beyond medical needs, understanding and responding to patients' emotional, social and spiritual needs will become an integral part of the profession.
- **Interdisciplinary collaboration**: Caring for Alzheimer's patients often requires the involvement of several professionals (occupational therapists, psychologists, physiotherapists, etc.). The nurse will often play the role of coordinator, ensuring smooth communication between the various professionals involved.
- **Education and awareness**: Faced with the stigma surrounding dementia, nurses will play a major role in educating the public, families and even other health professionals.
- **Clinical research**: With a disease as prevalent and debilitating as Alzheimer's, clinical research will be crucial. Nurses could play a more active role in research, whether it's implementing clinical trials or observing and documenting patients' symptoms and progress.
- **Defending patients' rights**: Guaranteeing the dignity, rights and well-being of Alzheimer's patients will

always be at the heart of the profession. This includes ethical issues such as informed consent, medical decision-making, etc.

- **Support for carers**: Given the stress and emotional burden associated with caring for Alzheimer's patients, the well-being and support of carers will be essential. This could take the form of additional training, support groups or mental health resources.

The Alzheimer's nursing profession is constantly evolving. Faced with the unique challenges posed by the disease, nurses will continue to adapt and innovate their approaches to offer the best possible care to their patients.

Chapter 34:
OUTLOOK FOR THE FUTURE
FOR ALZHEIMER CARE

Progress medical and therapeutic

Alzheimer's disease, as the most common form of dementia, has been the subject of much research over the years. Medical and therapeutic advances are crucial to improving patients' quality of life and, eventually, finding a cure. Here is an overview of recent advances in this field:

- **New drugs**: While the drugs currently available are mainly aimed at slowing the progression of symptoms, research is continuing into treatments that can halt or even reverse the progression of the disease.
- **Non-pharmacological therapies**: Interventions such as music therapy, art therapy, aromatherapy and animal therapy have shown promising results in improving mood, reducing anxiety and improving communication in Alzheimer's patients.
- **Early detection**: The ability to diagnose Alzheimer's disease at an early stage, even before symptoms appear, could enable treatment to begin earlier. Advances in brain imaging, biomarkers and genetic tests all point in this direction.
- **Gene therapy**: Research into genetic manipulation to treat or prevent Alzheimer's disease is still at an early stage, but it offers a promising way forward.
- **Vaccines**: Studies are underway to develop a vaccine against Alzheimer's disease that would specifically target the amyloid plaques or neurofibrillary tangles characteristic of the disease.

- **Technology**: The use of applications, therapeutic video games and virtual reality devices offers new ways of stimulating the brain, improving memory and slowing the progression of the disease.
- **Support for carers**: Recognising the enormous pressure on carers of Alzheimer's patients, new programmes and resources are being put in place to offer emotional, educational and practical support.
- **Lifestyle interventions**: Studies have shown that interventions focusing on diet, exercise and mental well-being can have a positive impact on cognitive health.
- **Research into risk factors**: Understanding why some people develop Alzheimer's and others don't is crucial. Recent research has explored factors such as inflammation, infections and imbalances in the gut microbiome.
- **Personalised treatment**: As in other areas of medicine, Alzheimer's research is moving towards more personalised treatments based on the specific needs of each patient.

The hope remains that medical and therapeutic advances will lead to more effective treatments, or even a cure, for Alzheimer's disease. The key lies in continued investment in research and innovation.

The evolution of training geriatric nurse

The evolution of geriatric nursing training reflects societal changes, medical advances and the growing recognition of the specific needs of the elderly. The care of the elderly has become increasingly complex, requiring a holistic approach that takes into account not only the medical aspects, but also the psychological, social and cultural dimensions of the elderly person's life.

- **Background**: Originally, nursing training was generalist, with little specialisation in geriatrics. Care for the elderly often focused on comfort care, with no specific approach.
- **Recognition of geriatrics as a speciality**: As Western societies aged and the needs of the elderly became more complex, the need for specialist training in geriatrics became clear.
- **Integrating multidisciplinarity**: Geriatric nursing training has gradually integrated the importance of working as part of a team with other professionals, such as geriatric doctors, social workers, occupational therapists, physiotherapists and psychologists.
- **Person-centred approach**: Curricula have evolved to emphasise a person-centred approach, valuing the autonomy, dignity and individual preferences of elderly patients.
- **Continuing and specialist training**: In addition to initial training, continuing and specialist training programmes in geriatrics have been set up, enabling nurses to keep abreast of best practice and the latest research in the field.
- **Incorporating technology**: Technology has become a key element of geriatric care, with training in the use of technological tools to assess, monitor and improve the quality of life of the elderly.
- **Emphasis on prevention**: The training also included the prevention of chronic diseases, health promotion and the importance of physical activity and a balanced diet for the well-being of the elderly.
- **Non-pharmacological approaches**: In response to concerns about over-medication of the elderly, geriatric nursing education has incorporated non-

pharmacological techniques to manage problems such as pain, agitation or insomnia.
- **Cultural skills**: As societies have become more diverse, training has incorporated the importance of understanding and respecting cultural, religious and ethnic differences in caring for the elderly.
- **Research and participation in nursing science**: Nurses are encouraged to participate in geriatric research, thereby contributing to the development of knowledge and best practice in this field.

The evolution of geriatric nursing training reflects the transformation of care for the elderly, recognising the uniqueness and complexity of this population and the importance of providing high-quality, respectful, person-centred care.

Hopes, challenges and opportunities on the horizon

The landscape of care for the elderly, particularly those with Alzheimer's and other forms of dementia, is constantly changing. As we look to the future, there are many hopes, challenges and opportunities on the horizon.

U23s :
- **Medical discoveries**: Hopes of finding a cure or more effective treatments for Alzheimer's are high, with continued progress in medical research.
- **Technology**: The increasing integration of technology offers the hope of improving the quality of life of patients, facilitating the work of carers and optimising the management and monitoring of care.
- **Holistic approaches**: A growing awareness of the importance of a holistic approach, integrating physical, mental, emotional and spiritual well-being,

offers the hope of more comprehensive, person-centred care.

- **Interdisciplinary collaboration**: The hope of greater collaboration between different healthcare professionals will enable patients to receive more comprehensive and effective care.

Challenges :

- **Demographics**: The increase in the elderly population poses challenges in terms of care capacity, infrastructure and resources.
- **Complex care**: As patients live longer, they often develop a number of chronic conditions, requiring complex management.
- **Costs**: The rising costs of healthcare, coupled with increasing demand, pose challenges in terms of funding and accessibility.
- **Lack of trained professionals**: The growing demand for healthcare professionals specialising in the care of the elderly and Alzheimer's sufferers often outstrips supply.

Opportunities :

- **Training and education**: With the growing awareness of the specific needs of elderly patients, there is an opportunity to broaden and improve the training of healthcare professionals in this area.
- **Technological innovations**: New technologies such as artificial intelligence, telemedicine and remote monitoring offer opportunities to transform the way care is delivered.
- **Alternative therapies**: There is a growing opportunity to integrate non-traditional therapeutic approaches, such as aromatherapy, music therapy or art therapy, into the care plan.
- **Working with families and volunteers**: Involving families and volunteers can be a valuable resource for

improving the quality of care and well-being of patients.

The future of care for people with Alzheimer's and the elderly in general is both promising and full of challenges. However, with the continued commitment of healthcare professionals, researchers, families and communities, there is solid hope of improving the quality of life of these individuals and overcoming the challenges that lie ahead.